MY WORLD'S BEST 100 RESTAURANTS 2019

METIN AR

DEDICATION

I dedicate this book to my lovely daughter, Esra Ar.

CONTENTS

ACKNOWLEDGMENTS

I thank my dear friend Reha Tanör for planting the idea for this undertaking in my mind and guiding me through this journey with his own great book "Restaurants and Tales". I thank Stefan Martens (see martens@gmail.com) for his perfect editing, and I'd also like to express my sincere gratitude to Chris Fielden (www.christopherfielden.com) for preparing the book for publishing. And last but not least, I thank Şule Şantarlı for the time and effort she put over the years to prepare the original text in Turkish.

Metin Ar

metinar@metinar.com

INTRODUCTION

In 2009, I started writing for a magazine about restaurants in different cities around the world. Every single one is an establishment that I liked; here, there are no places with negative reviews. Later, I started publishing these dispatches for a blog called Metin Ar Restaurant Writings (www.metinar.com/travel). Since then, I've continued to add to the blog, keeping it up to date in both English and Turkish. When I learned about the possibility of publishing a book with Amazon, I decided to convert the content into a book in both print and Kindle formats. And because I intend to update the book every year, readers will always have the opportunity to peruse the latest version.

Metin Ar

metinar@metinar.com

MY 15 FAVORITE RESTAURANTS

The results for 2018 are in. After deliberations among 900 jury members, Restaurant magazine and San Pellegrino have come up with the 50 best restaurants in the world.

The list is formed by jury members who each rank their 10 favorite eateries in order of preference, ultimately producing a list of 50. I can't keep myself to just 10 restaurants, so let me note my top 15, albeit in alphabetical order, rather than order of quality.

1. ARZAK (San Sebastian/ Spain) (31)
Paquita Arzak established Arzak in the 1960s, eventually bringing her son Juan Mari Arzak on board to work in the kitchen. Now 70, Juan Mari runs the show today, along with his daughter. Arzak got its first Michelin star in 1974, its second in 1978 and its third in 1989, making it the first three-star restaurant in Spain.

When Ferran Adria became famous 10 years ago, everybody lined up to criticize him for serving 30 to 40 portions. Juan Mari, however, called up Ferran and asked to see what he was

doing. After observing Ferran's work, Juan Mari said he had learned a lot from El Bulli's master and duly invited him to come to San Sebastian.

Soon, the two gastronomic titans became close friends, traveling to different places around the world together and trying different food. Their close friendship notwithstanding, they have different styles and tastes.

Arzak has two gastronomical menus, both of which mainly have meat – perhaps too much meat – instead of fish. I managed to get half portions for each of the courses, which allowed me to try 10 portions that actually amounted to two starters, a main course and a dessert. Now normally, restaurants with three Michelin stars don't allow you to mix and match like this, as they see it as beyond them, but Arzak isn't so snooty as to not offer such an option to its diners.

2. ATTICA (Melbourne/Australia) (20)

It's well-nigh impossible to find a seat at this Australian restaurant, which is among the cream of the crop near the top of the world's top 50 list. In the end, we had Mehmet Gürs' intervention to thank for allowing us to make a reservation, although it wasn't under the most ideal of circumstances: We had to be there at 6 p.m. – not my most preferred time – and out by 8:30 p.m. Attica has a set menu for all; the only possible alteration is to choose fish if you don't eat meat. Nonetheless, we reckoned that it would be impossible to come all the way to Melbourne and not go to Attica. The prices truly are astronomical, but boy was the food out of this world. It was the best meal I had in Melbourne, but more than that, if I were on the jury to vote for the world's best restaurant, I think I'd probably vote for Attica. We had a 12-course menu, 10 of which we enjoyed. I had no complaints because I opted to go meat-free, although my daughter did not. Ultimately, that meant that she had to dine out on fried ant (probably for the first and last time), which is consumed in Australia. If you're not interested in ingesting delicacies like this, it's a good idea to sometimes put a limit on the meat.

3. BLUE HILL (New York/USA) (12)

Blue Hill is about 50 minutes out of town by cab in Stone Barns at a ranch that was, interestingly, built by Rockefeller. Here, they grow all kinds of organic vegetables and raise pigs, chicken and small cows. I don't generally deign to eat eggs, but I definitely did here.

Everything looks good, smells nice and tastes even better, probably because of the fodder they use. All the meals, apart from the fish, are prepared with the freshest of ingredients that are produced right on the farm. Blue Hill's chef, Dan Barber, has been in charge of the kitchen since day one. You can enjoy a dinner at Blue Hill six days a week, while there is also an additional lunch service on Saturdays and Sundays. This being the United States, dinner begins as early as 5:30 p.m., so I recommend you make a reservation for as early in the evening as possible. More than that, try and go an hour early, because it's a lot of fun to spend time both in the town and the farm. (And don't be tardy about planning your trip to Blue Hill either: Reservations are a big problem at the restaurant, but if you send an email at least five or six weeks in advance and are flexible about time, you'll get results.)

A spacious and calm place with 10-meter-high ceilings, Blue Hill can host 50 people. Thankfully, the tables are spread out from one another, allowing you to chat comfortably. Blue Hill also has a splendid wine menu, which has offerings from all over the world at a good price. At your typical fine restaurant, the wines are priced at a wholesale price multiplied by around four; at Blue Hill, however, they only multiply this price by two, even though it's a top restaurant. More than that, you can order wines by the glass, giving you the opportunity to taste a different wine for every dish if you plan to try five or six different things. On top of that, all the waiters at Blue Hill are very knowledgeable about food and wine. And while most New York restaurants typically have a high circulation in terms of waiters, almost all of Blue Hill's wait staff have been there since the first day.

An Alumnus from the Obama Administration
The restaurant's chef, Dan Barber, also used to be on former U.S. President Barack Obama's Council on Fitness, Sports and Nutrition. In 2009, Barber was also selected as the best chef in New York by an independent jury, while Time also declared him one of the 100 most influential people that same year. Barber might be influential, but the farmers he sources his food from are even more influential – at least in terms for what makes it onto his menu. "I don't decide what to cook that day, farmers do. I form my menus according to the products farmers pick and I shape personal menus in line with our guests' requests."

4. DINNER BY HESTON London/England) (45)
Heston Blumenthal launched Dinner By Heston inside the Mandarin Oriental Hotel in London. I once had a lunch appointment with an important customer of mine and wanted to take him to the restaurant. But try as I might (twice, in fact), I couldn't land a booking for my preferred date. In my hour of need, I turned to İsa

Bal, the sommelier of the Fat Duck, Blumenthal's first restaurant, for help. İsa was able to open doors, and I finally went there with my guest.

The system at Dinner by Heston is different than that of the Fat Duck, as Blumenthal continues to serve a 17-course menu at his first location. For Dinner By Heston, it appears that he has employed his own right-hand person, Ashley Palmer, as executive chef. About 10-12 chefs cook in a tiny glass room that resembles an aquarium; it might make the cooks feel like they're in a fishbowl, but it allows you to watch your food being prepared.

Another great thing is that all of the dishes here are drawn from the cuisine of Medieval England. The menu includes the history of the dish, as well as further elaborate information about how it was cooked. Dinner By Heston has a simpler menu compared to the Fat Duck, but the beauty of this place is that it is open every single day, including Sundays. What's more, it has a great view of Hyde Park.

5. DISFRUTAR (Barcelona/Spain) (18)

Disfrutar is a restaurant belonging to three young, former employees of El Bulli: Mateu Casañas, Oriol Castro and Eduard Xatruch. The trio earned their first Michelin star in no time at all, but arrogance is nowhere to be seen when you take a look at the restaurant. Disfrutar has three different menus with 12, 18 and 25 courses. More than that, the staff can all rapidly shift gears from meat to fish. There are options to dine at either the table or at the bar, but I'm one of those who prefers the latter so that I'm able to watch as the meals are prepared and even chat with the chefs at times. I generally find the bar section quite interactive and fun but, of course, it depends on the restaurant...

In my opinion, Disfrutar reflects the Ferran Adria school better than any of its rivals. Unsurprisingly, Disfrutar is always full, so I'd advise you to make a reservation ahead of time – even a couple of months ahead of time. Nevertheless, you might have luck if you try and book for lunchtime.

Disfrutar separates the evening service into two sessions. The first service begins at around 7 p.m., while the second commences at around 9.30 p.m. But given that this is night-owl Spain, the second service typically draws more people – meaning that if you're more of an early bird, you might not have that many problems booking reservations for 7 p.m.

6. EL CELLER DE CAN ROCA (Girona/ Spain) (2)

A place with three Michelin stars, Can Roca is located about an hour northeast of Barcelona in beautiful Girona. Can Roca, the third best restaurant on this year's list, serves up classic fare. It's also a fraternal affair: Joan Roca is the chef, Joseph Roca is the sommelier and Jordi Roca, the youngest brother, is the pastry chef. The restaurant, which has a capacity for about 60 or 70 people, is in a very nice and modern building with pleasing architecture.

They have an option for an à la carte menu, but I would suggest trying the 12-portion menu, which is accompanied by very suitable and affordable wine. It's probably best to go there for lunch – a meal there is a five-and-a-half-hour event (I, for one, went for lunch at 1 p.m. and only managed to leave 6:30 p.m.), so that's something to consider if you don't want to finish dinner after midnight and then wonder how you're ever going to get to sleep.

7. ELEVEN MADISON PARK (New York/ USA) (4)

Eleven Madison Park was named the world's best restaurant in 2017. I wasn't impressed the first time I went there for lunch, but boy was I charmed by their dinner service the second time I went. From 7 p.m. to 11:30 p.m., our group of four had a wonderful meal. First of all, there is no menu here; instead, our waiter chatted with us to find out about what we like and don't like. Armed with this information, they prepared personal menus consisting of 15 dishes. I had fish, while my friends had meat and veggies. And all through the meal, chefs and waiters swung by our table to tell us the stories of each of our dishes. Moreover, there was a meaningful touch on every plate. It was just like a cabaret … It was most certainly an exciting and enjoyable dinner.

The place, which can host 50-60 people, boasts church-like high ceilings that create a sense of comfort. The tables are also distant from one another, which spares you some of the noise from the other tables. And in my humble opinion, the wine menu is also great. It's usually a tall order trying to find half-bottles of wine on the menu, but Eleven Madison Park is one of those rare places (it's also something that allows them to serve a number of good brands). We, for one, had a half-bottle of the famous and rare Petrus for, appropriately enough, half the price of a normal Petrus, although we also tried different wines with every dish.

8. LE BERNARDIN (New York/USA)
(26)

One of the first places that comes to mind when you say food and New York is Le Bernardin. Gilbert and Mathilde Le Coze opened the famous fish restaurant first in Paris in 1972 before raising the curtain on a second branch in New York 14 years later. Gilbert, who was also the chef, passed away shortly after the opening, giving way to Eric Ripert, one of his associates. Although the cuisine is French in origin, it is quite Americanized today.

In my opinion, Le Bernardin is the best fish restaurant in New York – everyone should eat there at least once. If you go there for lunch, you can have a beautiful fish menu in a very comfortable environment for a lower price than usual. Normally, I don't like the service of three-Michelin-star restaurants because of their attitude, but Le Bernardin is one such restaurant with three Michelin stars that has great service. Try to make reservations a week in advance.

9. MIKLA (Istanbul/Turkey) (44)

Mehmet Gürs' Mikla has finally cracked the top 50, coming in at number 44. When the rankings for 2019 come out, however, I imagine Mikla will move up the list. Gürs offers a three-course meal and a six-course one, one of which can be vegetarian.

Mikla's food is local, and nothing is frozen. The cooks, too, are always on their feet, as just seven cook for the 140 guests that dine from 6 p.m. to midnight.

The wine list is approved by Wine Spectator and features top Turkish varieties. Add in the best view in town, as well as perfect service, and you absolutely can't go wrong with Mikla.

10. MIRAZUR (Nice/France) (3)

France saves some of its best for last: Mirazur, the world's third-best restaurant, is located in Menton, the last town on the Côte d'Azur before you hit Italy. Heading up the restaurant is an Argentine chef, Mauro Colagreco, who cooks French dishes. If you want ironed cotton tablecloth like me, they'll immediately bring one to you. If you don't, you can eat at a wooden table as if you're at a kebab place. And naturally, given its location on the Riviera, it has an unreal view.

11. OSTERIA FRANCESCANA (Modena/ Italy) (1)

A place with three Michelin stars, the Osteria Francescana in Modena finally earned its rightful place as the best restaurant in the world in 2016, although it fell back to second in 2017. The restaurant's capacity, however, is as small as its reputation is big. The osteria has one dining room for 10 people, as well as another one for 20 people – ultimately meaning it's difficult to find a place at one of the individual tables.

If you do snag a place at this paragon of modern Italian cuisine, may I suggest you try the gastronomical menu. But if you're pressed for time, try three or four dishes. The dishes are served as small, non-fusion portions. Francescana goes for the minimal in its decoration, although it does have colorful walls. The restaurant is also located in an alley, which can cause problems, especially as the area is closed to traffic on the weekends, meaning you might need to stretch your legs a bit if you're arriving by car on Saturday or Sunday.

12. PIAZZA DUOMO (Alba/Italy) (16)

Listed as the 15th best restaurant of 2017, Piazza Duomo is not only Alba's most famous restaurant, but it is also one of the most expensive restaurants in Italy. Alba is a paradise of truffles. White truffles, which are more valuable than black truffles, are the star of the region. For this reason, I'd recommend you visit Alba in fall when white truffles are in season. Piazza Duomo is open throughout the year, but if you go to the restaurant sometime between October and December, you'll get the chance to taste the unique white truffle. A place with three Michelin stars, Piazza Duomo is located on the second floor of a building right in front of the city's main church. They have an à la carte menu, but I recommend the gastronomical one.

13. STEIERECK (Vienna/Austria) (14)

Located inside a city park in Vienna is Steiereck, the world's 10th best restaurant. The couple that runs the place don't open on weekends, so you'll need to make reservations in advance. Steiereck offers a great view of the surrounding park thanks to its floor-to-ceiling windows, making you feel like you're eating in the center of a garden full of beautiful flowers and trees. Steiereck has a tasting menu that you can order for either lunch or dinner. The restaurant can prepare the menu, one of which is fish-based and the other meat-based, depending on your preferences. One useful thing about Steiereck is that they bring cards written in both English and German explaining the dishes – it's a great idea given that many waiters outside the United States have less than fluent English. And to enhance the experience, they provide a small stand on the table so that you can read as you eat. You can even take the card with you if you're interested in saving the recipe. All in all, Steiereck is a wonderful experience.

14. TEST KITCHEN (Cape Town/South Africa) (50)
At Test Kitchen, half of the restaurant is a kitchen – there's just a counter that divides this large place in two. On one side, they host guests, while on the other, they're cooking the dishes. The cooks put the meals they've prepared on the counter, the waiters take the dishes and serve them – it's very simple and intimate. It's a relaxing place that's decorated with very nice objects, while it also has a very rich wine menu. You can find beautiful wines from other countries, as well as the best examples of South African wine. If you like, you can take your own wine with you. Whatever the case, you should come prepared for a big meal; it takes three hours in the afternoon and four in the evening (but as someone who's tried both, let me note that the evening menu is preferable).

Test Kitchen opens its doors at 7 p.m. for dinner and continues all the way to 11 p.m. It's a long dinner that calls for an empty stomach, so I suggest you skip lunch. If you're a vegetarian or prefer fish/meat, you can let them know in advance so that they can organize their menu in accordance with your preferences. (I, for one, really enjoyed the vegetable and fish menu.) Test Kitchen has adapted a fusion-dominant culinary approach in which they use fruit in a number of dishes – I especially liked their sweet-and-sour sauce that was made from fruit. They also like to serve their fish and seafood undercooked, while the last three courses are cheese, dessert and fruit.

15. TICKETS (Barcelona/Spain) (32)

Tickets was introduced to Barcelona's food lovers by the brother of Ferran Adria, the founder of the legendary El Bulli. All the dishes (many of which have migrated from El Bulli here), whether on the 20- to 25-course menu or the à la carte one, consist of just two or three bites.

Finding a seat is next to impossible at Tickets, which only accepts online reservations. The maximum reservation period is also just two months, but if you can arrange your plans two months in advance, you can take your chance for a meal at Tickets. Although it's a simple restaurant, the food is extraordinary. The place opens at around 7 in the evening and continues until midnight.

ALBA

There are mushrooms and then there are mushrooms. Deemed one of the world's most valuable edible fungi, "white truffles" are found in few areas of the world, one of which is Alba, a small town in Italy's Piedmont region that's south of Milan. On this front, the word "found" is more than apt, for the white truffle defies cultivation, making it more like a precious metal than a crop.

Every year, truffle lovers descend on Alba, a town that I've had the pleasure of visiting seven times in the past. It's a place I love, so let me share some of my previous experiences with you.

WHEN'S THE BEST TIME TO VISIT?
You can visit Alba from the beginning of September until January, but the best move is to plan your visit for autumn, particularly in November – that's when the town hosts its annual White Truffle Fair to coincide with the abundance of truffles. Beware, though, that accommodation fills up fast, so it's best to book ahead, particularly if you're planning on seeing the town over the weekend amid the rest of the world's truffle lovers. But if you're too late to visit during the height of truffle season, consider March or April, when Alba is also lovely.

HOW DO YOU GO HUNT FOR TRUFFLES?
It's no surprise that everyone wants to grow something like a truffle, given that it's sometimes valued at a whopping 3,000 euros per kilogram. Mother Nature, however, won't allow you to grow them; what's more,

it's hard to predict where and when to find them. Because of that, you'll need to follow the nose of a trained dog or pig to help you discover these edible underground "diamonds."

But while pigs continue to be used in France, their swine compatriots are no longer used over the border in Italy. That's because pigs are wilder than dogs, meaning they can damage the truffle – as well as the hunter. When pigs find truffles, it's all the hunter can do to pull off the pig, lest it seize the prized fungus for itself. With a dog, by contrast, the task of pulling it away is comparatively easier. That's why you might even come across Italian hunters without a right hand after they lost it to a pig intent on enjoying a truffle or two.

Due to an increase in the number of hunting accidents – and especially given the number of hunters who lost their hands – Italy's Parliament outlawed the use of pigs in truffle hunts, even if the animals are more adept at scouting out the fungi than dogs.

I've gone hunting for truffles three times, and I can safely say it's a gruelling experience! Truffles are found in wooded areas, particularly within about 100 to 150 centimeters from the roots of oak trees.

At various hotels in Alba, you can agree on a price with a truffle hunter before setting off for a hunt. In general, the best time to hunt is between 5 or 6 in the morning, but the evening sometimes works as well.

Whatever you do, a well-trained dog is a must – along with a hunter who knows how to lead the dog to find the truffles. It's funny – the hunters of other game typically like to overstate the success of their exploits, but truffle hunters are exactly the opposite. If you ask them how their hunt went, they'll probably tell you it was a fiasco! After all, the rarer and less plentiful the truffle, the higher the price.

After you, your dog and your truffle hunter find your quarry, it's time to remove the truffles from the ground and clean off the soil and mud with a brush. After that, you clean them again with a wet towel, followed by a wipe-down with a dry towel. Whatever you do, just don't wash them with water! After they've dried, you put them in a jar to preserve the flavor. But once they've been removed from the ground, truffles, whether of the black or white variety, must be consumed within a week at most; otherwise, they will lose their flavor.

WHAT'S THE BEST WAY TO EAT TRUFFLES?
When it comes time to eat, may I suggest you shave the truffles with a shaver at the table as this method is sure to give off the fungi's inviting aroma – the most important thing when eating truffles.

Truffles go best with risotto and pasta. If the harvest was abundant, black truffles are often preserved in jars of olive oil. Such an olive oil goes great with salads and pasta, although it's best with hot dishes, since the aroma is so much more intense.

WHAT ARE THE BEST RESTAURANTS FOR TRUFFLES IN ALBA?

LA CIAU DEL TORNAVENTO
La Ciau Del Tornavento has a menu that offers a wide range of truffle dishes. It also boasts a spectacular wine cellar, which allows patrons to enjoy almost every class

and taste of Italian and French wines.

What makes La Ciau a special treat – particularly for lunch – is its mesmerising view from atop a hill. If you choose to have a pleasant meal at the restaurant, give my regards to the grand chef Maurilio, who also doubles as the owner of this fine establishment.

TRATTORIA LA POSTA
My second suggestion is a place that is also perfect for lunch.

LA LIBERA
The third place I can recommend is La Libera, a long-time fixture in Alba. Close to the city center, La Libera is a good choice for lunch or dinner.

PIAZZA DUOMO
One of the town's most famous and exclusive restaurants is Piazza Duomo. It's not only Alba's most famous restaurant, it's also one of the most expensive restaurants in Italy. Listed as the world's 15th best restaurant in 2017, it also has three Michelin stars. Piazza Duomo is located on the second floor of a building right in front of the city's main church. The service might be a bit slow, but there are so many surprising appetizers that you're likely to spend at least three hours dining. They have an à la carte menu, but I recommend the gastronomical one.

Piazza Duomo is open throughout the year, but if you go to the restaurant sometime between October and December, you'll get the chance to taste the unique white truffle. In short, I can't recommend

Piazza Duomo enough.

VILLA D'AMELIA

Villa d'Amelia is the best choice for accommodation, although it also features an excellent restaurant for dinner.

A FEW SPECIAL TRUFFLE RECIPES

In the mood for something with truffles? Then here's a pair of simple recipes. If you want to save a bit and opt for cheaper truffles, allow me to recommend summer truffles, which are available between June and September. Before you start, though, make sure you're ready with a special truffle shaver.

TRUFFLE WITH EGGS/TRUFFLE OMELETTE:

Truffles pair best with eggs, which blend well with the fungi's intense flavor and aroma.

Break an egg in a saucepan and heat it up until the white of the egg is well-done but the yolk is still rare. Before serving, sprinkle on a good-quality salt.

Repeat the process for everyone who's eating.

Once the eggs are on the table, everyone can take the shaver and grate the truffle onto their eggs. Accompany this simple but excellent meal with some freshly baked bread.

If you have more guests coming, you can, alternatively, beat 10 eggs and add them to a pan that has been greased with a bit of truffle oil. But don't leave it on for too long, as there's no need for the omelette to be well-done. To add to the aroma, you can add a couple drops of truffle oil to the plates before serving. Like the straight egg option before, shave black or white truffles onto the omelette before eating – doing so at the table will intensify the flavor and smell.

TRUFFLE SPAGHETTI:

Cook some fresh pasta or spaghetti lightly for two or three minutes, whisking it in truffle oil. Remove the pasta from the heat, allowing everyone to add their own truffle shavings.

If the white truffle's cost of 2,000 to 2,500 euros a kilo is a bit too rich for your blood, summer truffles cost a more inexpensive 150 to 200 euros. The flavor of black truffles is not as intense as the white, but the lower costs means there will be more shavings to go around for your meal.

*A tip: Once you've shaved the truffles so much that you can't grate them anymore, you can put the leftovers in a jar and add some butter. Keep the jar in the deep freezer so that you can enjoy them whenever you want – after all, it's what Alba restaurants do when truffles are out of season.

AMALFI AND CAPRI

"DOLCE FAR NIENTE"

If you're still at a loss about where to spend vacation next year, look no further than southern Italy's Amalfi coast and the Island of Capri – the perfect place for a week-long getaway.

If you're interested in a one-week sojourn on the Amalfi Coast and Capri, let me tell you a bit about my trip to the area. But right off the bat, a caveat emptor: It's not a particularly budget-friendly holiday, but you could always cut down on the length of your stay; it's totally up to you!

It might be busy, but the best time to take a trip is July or August, when the weather is unlikely to throw up any nasty surprises. All you have to do is go, relax and enjoy the sun.

CUTTING DOWN ON COSTS

A trip to Amalfi and Capri isn't the cheapest vacation, but there are some ways to lighten the burden on your wallet. For one, there's no need to insist that your hotel room has a sea view – there will be plenty of chances to soak in the sea, and foregoing a view from your room will certainly save you from overspending. There are some other tricks while dining as well: Consider skipping out on both breakfast and lunch and just opting for brunch. Not only will it help you keep down the calorie intake amid all the wonderful food on offer, but it will also save you a bit of cash. Come dinner, you can try and avoid more of the priciest wines to cut back on cost as well.

After arriving in Naples by plane, grab a taxi – there's no reason to rent a car, as a cab will be more than enough to reach your destination. Take the road to Ravello, a town situated in the hills. The trip, which you should take without entering Naples proper or the coastal road, takes about 55 minutes using highways and other roads.

From 350-meter-high Ravello, you can survey all that is before you, including Amalfi, Positano and Capri. There are plenty of hotels in this small town, but only two hotels – Palazzo Avino and Hotel Caruso – that are really worthy of a night's stay. We stayed in the town for a night, enjoying a meal at Palazzo Avino and sleeping at Hotel Caruso.

Palazzo Avino's restaurant, Rossellinis, boasts two Michelin stars, a fantastic selection of wines and a well-regarded menu. You can select something to eat from the à la carte menu, but if you are dedicated to food, then plan to come to Rossellinis at 8:30 p.m., open a nice bottle of wine, and let yourself go with the flow of the menu until 11 p.m.

RAVELLO MUSIC FESTIVAL

The Ravello Music Festival starts in June and runs until mid-September, offering concerts every Friday and Saturday and, occasionally, other weekdays. You'll have a chance to sample the performances by different musicians each time; sometimes, it might be an orchestra and sometimes, it might just be a soloist.

Alternatively, you could go for a quick dinner and watch a Saturday night concert at the Ravello Music Festival from a terrace with a sea view. A word to the wise, though: The concert can be popular, so book a seat for the performance when you reserve your hotel room. Otherwise, you might find yourself stuck in the back rows or, worse, without any seat at all. Because the concert starts at 9:30 p.m., it's best to plan to eat at 7 and finish by 9 to make it to the performance on time. In such a case, may I recommend that you select your meal from the à la carte menu. After that, sit back and enjoy the sunset – but things will be even better if your concert under the stars also features a full moon!

On my last trip to Ravello, I hadn't booked a seat at the concert and, what's more, I hadn't even eaten lunch. As such, I abandoned myself to the joys of Rossellinis' gastronomic menu and delicious wine. During one of my previous visits, however, I did get the chance to watch the concert and the mesmerizing view. Needless to say, it was wonderful in every sense of the word.

The next day, head for a sightseeing tour of Ravello, including the local museum, if you so desire. Soon, however, the time will come to decide whether to head for Amalfi or Positano, two charming towns on the Amalfi Coast. If you choose Amalfi, you can stay at Santa Caterina – a place whose food is so exquisite you need never eat anywhere else in town, including lunch (provided that you make sure you have a light lunch, of course).

Santa Caterina is a newly restored, luxurious hotel in a historical building on a cliff above the sea. The hotel has two elevators inside the mountain that whisk you down to the sea, where you can find sunbeds, beach umbrellas and waiter service. Although the coast here does not have any sandy beach, there is a beautifully located pier.

If you opt for Positano instead, I suggest you try the Hotel San Pietro di Positano. After some breakfast, a chance to catch up on reading under an umbrella, a swim, a sailing trip with the hotel's boat and light lunch, prepare for dinner at 7 p.m. in the hotel's restaurant, a location that sports a Michelin star and a great service team. The grandchildren of the founder run the hotel, while the waiters are veterans who have been working at the establishment since the age of 20. Everybody at the restaurant treats you as if you were staying at their very house. The food and the wine are remarkable, but most importantly, they never try to take advantage of their customers – something that doesn't necessarily ring true for many seaside establishments around the world.

CONVENIENT TRANSPORT

Hotels in Positano have boats that can take you directly to Capri. And if you're in the mood to swim immediately, board the boat with your swimwear on; that way, you can dive into the waters of Capri as soon as you arrive while the hotel brings your luggage to your room.

Beyond the Hotel San Pietro, however, I wouldn't recommend any other restaurants in Positano. Even if you fail to find accommodation at the accompanying hotel, enjoying a meal there is a must, especially the risotto or macaroni with seafood, grilled fish and a light dessert.

Soon, though, it's time to move on again. As you head for Capri, plan to stay at least four nights. In terms of accommodation, you could never go wrong with the Hotel Capri Palace.

The Capri Palace has a two-star restaurant called L'Olivo, which is a great choice for breakfasts and a couple of dinners. They serve phenomenal wine, including some Turkish wines.

The best thing about the hotel is that it is located on the highest point of the island, giving it panoramic views. Luckily, however, it takes just five minutes to get to the Capri Palace's beach club, Il Riccio ("sea urchin") with transport provided by the hotel. As a hotel guest, a sunbed and umbrella will automatically be reserved for your use – which is a good thing, given that many people come from outside the hotel for a swim and the fare on offer. Il Riccio's food is sea-heavy – in fact, it's the only thing on the menu. By all means, eat lunch here, but I suggest you avoid filling up on food too much during the day, lest you lose your appetite for the dinner at L'Olivo.

While L'Olivo and Il Riccio are perfect for dinner, you should set aside at least one evening for supper at Aurora in town, where they have the lightest pizza I have ever sampled, a dish known as "water pizza." Sit outside and engage in a bit of people-watching at this lively place, which is run by a mother and her daughter. The daughter's name is Mia while the mother, naturally, is Mamma, giving us – you guessed it – "Mamma Mia!"

CHAMBER OF SIN

The Hotel Capri Palace also has a chamber of sin – a room full of delicious chocolates and desserts. The chamber of sin also serves fruit, but when you see the desserts, you can't possibly think about anything else.

Entry costs 20 euros, but it's up to you as to how to exit: The price of admission gives you the chance to dig into anything and everything, so you should bear in mind the potential for weight gain if you're operating under the impression that you have to eat everything just because you paid for it. Just dreaming about the desserts will get you salivating, but you might wake up wondering how you're going to lose all those calories…

AMSTERDAM

THE CITY OF CANALS THAT HAS BECOME A GASTRONOMICAL HEAVEN

Amsterdam is already one of the most beautiful cities in the world, but it might soon be adding another feather to its cap – namely, that of becoming a gastronomical getaway. It's all thanks to double taxation agreements that have prompted many umbrella companies to set up shop here.

If you're paying taxes in the Netherlands, you're not obliged to pay taxes in your home country as per the terms of the double taxation agreements. Nevertheless, companies engaged in such a practice can still get caught in their own country if the latter says you're running an inactive company to avoid taxes. To prevent this, many companies hold executive board meetings in Amsterdam once a year. Ergo, I have been going to Amsterdam for four years to attend the executive board meeting of an international company.

The meetings usually last two days, but if you add the travel time, I end up getting a four-day trip to Amsterdam. All senior executives have to attend the meetings, which brings together around 40-50 people – all of whom have to be reimbursed for accommodation and dining. And with some companies organizing two executive board meetings a year, there are plenty of high-powered and hungry business leaders in the city of canals all the time. Cue a new trend, in which many beautiful restaurants have started to open up over the past decade to satisfy businesspeople coming for meetings. It all means that

Amsterdam's restaurant scene – as well as the prices – have become richer.

It's a similar story in London, New York and Dubai, where executives appointed from other countries lose the habit of eating at home and start dining out over the three to five years they spend away from home (sometimes on their own dime, and sometime on their company's). Moreover, these companies host many guests as well. In any case, Amsterdam is now mentioned in the same breath as this trio – although there are sure to be more additions to the list due to Brexit, as many banks and finance companies relocate from London to elsewhere in Europe.

And it wasn't just businesspeople from around the world that were descending on Amsterdam but restaurateurs as well. To cater to the increased demand, many came to open new restaurants, while Dutch chefs also made their way back home to open new places. In short, Amsterdam has become a city of attraction. Beyond that, good hotels have started to rent out their own restaurants, which is the reason why Amsterdam's hotel restaurants don't have that cold and negative atmosphere shared by most such eateries. Each one is owned by a chef, meaning ambitious and hardworking chefs are in abundance in the city.

Over the past couple of years, I've had the chance to visit about 40 restaurants in Amsterdam. Of these, eight are really worth mention. Some of these eateries are expensive, and some are not. Naturally, the prices rise as the number of Michelin stars rise. So let me run the rule over them, proceeding, as always, in alphabetical order. And do let me know what you think by emailing metinar@metinar.com!

THE MOST DELICIOUS CLAMS EVER

Amsterdam is great for a wide variety of fresh seafood. When you're in town, may I suggest you try the clams as well. This delicious shellfish isn't particularly popular in Turkey, where it's imported as frozen food in fairly small quantities. In Amsterdam, however, the clams are huge! Besides, they're fresh every day, cooked in an oven in its shell and served with sauce on the side.

BORD EAU

Bord Eau is a French restaurant situated in a five-star hotel by the canal. The place doesn't draw many people during lunch hour, so the management decided to change things up by creating cheaper lunch menus with three courses. Even such inexpensive fare doesn't disappoint, as Bord Eau always serves everything like a restaurant with two Michelin stars. Waiters with gloves, butter and bread, chic presentations, little petit fours after the meal, chocolate – it's all there... And because the restaurant is in the city, you can walk there if you want to. More than that, it has a wonderful view of the canal! Amsterdam's canals are the equivalent of our streets, so you get to observe the city's life while you're dining at Bord Eau. If you have time for lunch, make sure to give this place a try.

BRIDGES

As its name suggests, Bridges is a restaurant in a neighborhood with many bridges. Like Bord Eau, it's a nice place by the canal that gives you the opportunity to watch Amsterdam's little boats pass by as you take it all in from the window. They also have a standard tasting menu, which is both economical and appealing, given that you never get a chance to try more than three different things when you order from the main menu. Nevertheless, I wouldn't recommend the tasting menu at Bridges. After all, the dishes on the main menu are beautifully designed like paintings. If you're not eating alone, you can order a number of different dishes with friends and feel as if you're eating in an art gallery. Bridges also has a good wine menu. If possible, make a reservation for a table by the window.

SALADS INSTEAD OF BREAD

Who can pass up fresh, warm bread? It's easy to lose oneself in a little bit of butter, olive oil and fresh, warm bread, but if you dig into that before the actual meal arrives, you'll hardly have any appetite for when the actual meal arrives. So give a pass on the bread and go for a salad instead.

CIEL BLUE

Ciel Blue is an authentic French restaurant located on the rooftop of a Japanese hotel somewhat outside the city center. The French chef at Ciel Blue, which sports two Michelin stars, has prepared a fantastic menu – particularly the tasting menu – for the place. The seabass, for one, is presented wonderfully here. I can easily pronounce Ciel Blue a gastronomical paradise. The restaurant doesn't have a canal view like the previous restaurants, but you can see the beautiful lights of the city in the distance. The Chinese and Japanese restaurants located in the same hotel also have a Michelin star each – giving the hotel four Michelin stars! The Chinese and Japanese restaurants, however, are not located well inside the hotel and have no view and no light. Not the best restaurants, I'd say.

SKYLOUNGE AMSTERDAM

There's a Hilton Hotel right next to the train station in Amsterdam. Actually, the hotel belongs to Hilton's sub brand DoubleTree By Hilton, which has better rates. That means that when you have to shell out 600 euros for a room in the normal Hilton, you can get a DoubleTree room at Hilton quality for a mere 300 euros. The best part of this Hilton is that there's a bar and a restaurant on the rooftop – the Hilton Sky Lounge, a great place that's open from 5 p.m. to midnight. The lounge has a panoramic view of Amsterdam, including the city's canals, train stations and churches. Even better, you can go there without a reservation. Everyone, from businesspeople to locals, loves to hang out there. Even if you're only in town for a day, I recommend you spend at least an hour at SkyLounge Amsterdam.

RIJKS

Rijks is located inside the peerless Rijksmuseum. If you're planning to make a reservation, keep in mind that there are two restaurants inside the museum. One is the Rijks café, which serves good food during the museum's visiting hours, and the other is the Rijks Restaurant, which has a Michelin star and is the place I want to recommend. You can access the restaurant, which has separate working hours, from the outside. You might not consider doing it elsewhere, but go and order five dishes at the Rijks since the portions are very small. Their cheese plates are delicious as well, so if you're a person who loves cheese as much as I do, you can order three dishes, a cheese plate and a cheese soufflé prepared with slightly sweet cheese. The restaurant serves lunch and dinner, and the none-too-expensive prices for both are the same.

LA RIVE

Located inside the Amstel Hotel, La Rive is a wonderful French restaurant with two Michelin stars. It has its own entrance outside the hotel, as well as one inside the hotel. Amstel Hotel is built on top of a canal, which gives La Rive a beautiful view of the wooden boats that pass by every now and then – in fact, your feet are almost below sea level since the restaurant is downstairs. Its watery address even gives you the option of arriving in style by boat, if you so desire. The chef appears to change from time, but the menu largely stays the same. Just like Bord Eau, the place isn't particularly crowded at lunchtime, while they even have a separate – and cheaper – lunch menu. Ultimately, La Rive is a place I've known for a decade and a half, and I can assure you that it will never disappoint.

VERMEER

Like La Rive, Vermeer is inside a hotel in central Amsterdam, although it also has an entrance of its own. This place has one Michelin star, but I imagine the time is coming when they will get a second star and a place in the top 100 list. Vermeer is my favorite restaurant in Amsterdam, but I think its inevitable second star will probably hurt the pocketbook a bit, as the place is already becoming more expensive by the day. Sometimes, restaurants increase their prices so much that I stop going, and I'm afraid that Vermeer's on this path too. So what's the moral of the story? Go before the prices skyrocket. Nonetheless, if I were to go to Amsterdam for a day, I'd still opt for Vermeer – after all, its scallop dish is delicious.

WOLF ATELIER

Owned by a chef named Wolf, this restaurant is located on the top floor of a shed by the canal with, you will not be surprised to learn, a great view of the waterways. Accessed by a metal staircase, Wolf Atelier has an open kitchen that allows you to watch everything from your seat. It isn't a very large place and features about seven or eight people in the kitchen and a similar number of servers. Wolf doesn't have a star and the prices are fairly inviting. The limited menu changes every day, as the restaurant decides to cook their meals based on what they can find daily. Naturally, that means you order off a printed A4 piece of paper rather than a luxurious menu. Whatever the case, you can smell the bread they cook in the oven the moment you step foot in the restaurant. When I'm in Amsterdam, I like to find some flounder from the English Channel and wild salmon from the North Sea – two dishes that Wolf Atelier does well. The wine list is also simple and affordable.

BARCELONA

Several years ago, world-famous chef Ferran Adria's restaurant El Bulli was a roaring success. Many chefs downed their tools to rush and learn about his understanding of molecular cuisine. Ferran, an intriguing personality and a gastronomic genius, has long since drawn the curtains on El Bulli, but those who have worked with him or adopted his ways now dominate the restaurant scene in Barcelona.

There's Ferran's understanding of molecular cuisine, the école he pioneered, Salvador Dali's influence on him, as well as his attempts to adapt the great surrealist's style of art to his cuisine. And then, of course, there is his masterpiece, El Bulli, which was named restaurant of the year several times ... A week before El Bulli closed its doors for good, I dined there and wrote about my experience. At El Bulli, upward of 60-70 chefs worked with him, but just a few received a wage; that's because chefs from around the world interned, so to say, just so that they could learn from his unique style. Because Ferran didn't know a word of English, he only selected applicants who spoke Spanish in the beginning. The selection process continued like this for a while until people advised him to change his approach: "Spanish is your criteria in selecting chefs, but you're losing brilliant chefs because of it! We'll handle the translation – just put the Spanish-only prerequisite aside." That talk changed things, as Ferran subsequently began to accept English-speaking chefs at El Bulli.

Just imagine: Important chef who were famous at home were applying to work alongside Ferran Adria as an assistant at El Bulli. Chefs who were accepted would leave everything behind and work as apprentices for six months. And because they were only apprentices, they might have just spent half a year peeling potatoes! Nevertheless, all the chefs did whatever it took in exchange for a piece of Ferran's wisdom. This part of the story is quite familiar to anyone who is fond of tasting dishes from talented chefs in famous restaurants around the world.

The really interesting story, however, began after Ferran closed El Bulli!

BARCELONA IS ROCKING

In recent times, Ferran's co-workers and other chefs who have matured at his school have started opening restaurants in Barcelona that reflect his understanding of cuisine. Some chefs have taken this step on their own, while some have formed teams to open the doors of new restaurants where they work their magic.

The only appropriate way to describe what these young chefs have been doing is to say they've been "rocking" the city for the past three or four years, having had the chance to combine their passion for cooking with the privilege of being Ferran's student. Continuing the greater master's legacy, these talented chefs have been leading a new trend; some chefs cook exactly like Ferran, while others have interpreted the chef d'école with their own touch. However, they all have one thing in common: the ability to "surprise."

Most of the dishes come in small portions, but Ferran will let you in on a little secret as to why it's more than fine to have portions that can be devoured in just two bites: "You'll admire the first bite, try the second and get bored by the third." With portions as small as this, menus can run as high as 20 or even 40 dishes.

With the movement in Barcelona catching my attention, I visited some marvelous restaurants to get a better taste of their dishes. Below, you can read about my experiences at 10 restaurants, all of which are from Ferran's école (seven of these belong to Ferran's students, while the remainder have been opened by followers). Avid readers know that I list in alphabetical order, but I've dispensed with tradition just this time and put the restaurants in the order of my own acclaim. If you ever find yourself at one of these restaurants, please let me know what you think.

THOSE YOUNG CHEFS AND THEIR RESTAURANTS!

Some of the places belonging to "Ferran's Kids," as we may call them, are organized like a bar, while others have traditional table settings. Anyway, as you sit at a stool in the former, you receive small portions of food from a man speaking broken English who tells you about the dish in front of you. Some other places, meanwhile, write the ingredients and the recipes on a piece of paper, recounting the story of a two-bite dish at great length. But whatever they do, all the places always do their job with gusto…

DISFRUTAR

It's been more than a year since the opening of Disfrutar, a restaurant belonging to three young, former employees of El Bulli: Mateu Casañas, Oriol Castro and Eduard Xatruch. The trio earned their first

Michelin star in no time at all, but arrogance is nowhere to be seen when you take a look at the restaurant. Disfrutar has three different menus with 12, 18 and 25 courses. More than that, the staff (all of whom, incidentally, have a good command of English) are able to rapidly shift gears from meat to fish when informed. There are options to dine at either the table or at the bar, but I'm one of those who prefers the latter so that I'm able to watch as the meals are prepared and even chat with the chefs at times. I generally find the bar section quite interactive and fun but, of course, it depends on the restaurant...

In my opinion, Disfrutar reflects the Ferran Adria school better than any of its rivals. Like all the restaurants mentioned below, Disfrutar is always full, so I'd advise you to make a reservation ahead of time – even a couple of months ahead of time! But here's a tip: it's way easier to find a place during lunchtime.

Interestingly, you have to spare three hours to eat because evening service is usually separated into two sessions at Spanish restaurants. The first service begins at around 7 p.m., with the second at around 9.30 p.m. This being Spain, the land of the late diners, the second service tends to attract a higher demand. Such Spanish tendencies, however, are a boon to those of us who are used to having dinner early, since it ensures that making reservations for 7 p.m. is comparatively easy.

Disfrutar boasts any number of marvelous "surprises," all of which are distinct to Ferran's école: An almond is not an almond, and an olive is not an olive...

TICKETS

Following Disfrutar is Tickets. According to critics, Tickets is the best restaurant in Barcelona. It was introduced to the city's food lovers by Ferran Adria's brother, who is currently receiving help from the master chef himself. Offering the same dishes as El Bulli, Tickets provides menus, whether of the 20- to 25-course or the à la carte variety, consisting of just two or three bites. And like other top-notch places, finding a seat is almost impossible.

Tickets only accepts online reservations. The maximum reservation period is also just two months (unlike El Bulli, which used to take reservations a year in advance). Although it's a simple restaurant, the food is extraordinary. The place opens at around 7 in the evening and continues until midnight.

DOS PALILLOS

Dos Palillos is a fusion of Japanese, Vietnamese, Chinese, Thai and Spanish cuisine that seats just 25 people. Albert Raurich, who worked with Ferran Adria, designed the restaurant with a three-cornered sushi bar, while the fourth corner opens up to the kitchen, where you can observe the preparation of your dish, every step of the way. Meals are prepared at both the bar and the kitchen, although it is mandatory to sit at the bar to eat. À la carte and other menu choices are available at the restaurant.

So what does a fusion of Asian and Spanish cuisine produce? For one, dishes with raw meat and fish cooked rare. Dos Palillos also has an extensive wine list of Spanish and international offerings that are all priced reasonably.

LASARTE

Probably Barcelona's most expensive restaurant, Lasarte has little connection to Ferran Adria apart from the fact that they use some of his style in their dishes. The owner of the place is Martin Berasategui, a chef who also owns a restaurant with three Michelin stars in San Sebastian. As you would expect, Lasarte is influenced by Basque cuisine, and the dishes are as delicious as they are at Berasategui's restaurant in San Sebastian. The famous chef is not currently at Lasarte – which has two Michelin starts – but he is most certainly the mastermind behind the food. The dishes include fruits and flowers, and even a bit of butter. Berasategui's restaurant in San Sebastian even has toothbrushes and toothpaste in the bathrooms – a detail which I really liked and a detail which has been replicated by Lasarte.

The place, mind you, is expensive, as is the wide-ranging wine menu. Still, if you want to reward yourself or let go for a day, Lasarte is the place to dine.

Though the restaurant is huge, Lasarte only has room for 20 people to sit – the result of a decision to provide a comfortable place for diners to chat and create a place with less interaction between the tables. Ultimately, its snow-white, unwrinkled napkins and ironed and clean tablecloths stand out – not to mention the waiters who are always eager to help whenever you lift your head up from your dish… In short, everything is perfect…

HOJA SANTA

There are two chefs in the kitchen of Hoja Santa: Albert Adrià and Paco Méndez. Hoja Santa is not in a frequently visited place in town, meaning it's easier to find a place during lunchtime. Nevertheless, the restaurant is pretty crowded at noon on Friday and Saturday. Hoja Santa blends Mexican and Spanish cuisine in a fusion of the former with Ferran Adria's style, although that doesn't mean that the dishes are out-of-this-world spicy, as you might expect from Mexican cuisine. Still, beans are in abundant supply. Again, the portions are small, while there are also little "surprises." You can dine either at the bar or at the table.

DOS CIELOS

Located on top of a hotel, Dos Cielos is a nice restaurant owned by twin chefs from El Bulli, Javier and Sergio Torres. The chefs look so much alike that you feel like you've had a little too much to drink, too early. If you go to the restaurant as two or three people, eating at the bar will be more fun, as it provides an interactive dining experience that I really enjoy. With a view from the top, a satisfactory wine menu and Ferran touches, Dos Cielos is definitely a restaurant I'd recommend.

CINC SENTITS

Number seven on the list is Cinc Sentits. It might not be from the Ferran Adria school, but it operates according to a similar style. Owned by Jordi and Amelia Artal, "Cinc Sentits" means "five senses" – so it's no surprise that they use senses like smelling and hearing in most of their dishes. Perhaps readers will remember: I mentioned a similar presentation while writing about my experiences at the Fat Duck. At the latter, they create an atmosphere according to what you order. For example, as you're eating seafood, the establishment's iPod plays wave sounds as a spray dispenses the freshening smell of the sea. It all means it's not just your taste but other senses as well that get addressed. The difference at Cinc Sentits, though, is that they create this atmosphere for almost every dish.

MOMENTS

Moments, located in the Mandarin Oriental Hotel, is a Ferran Adria restaurant to the T. The luxurious restaurant is owned by Ferran's brother. Moments is a chic, centrally located and tremendously expensive restaurant. They offer menus of four or five portions. Unsurprisingly given that it is located in the Mandarin Oriental Hotel, Moments has turned itself into a hotel restaurant, in contrast to the other restaurant owned by Ferran's brother, Tickets, which is more like a tapas bar. Like some of the others on this list, it's easier to score a place for lunch at Moments.

ABAC

Every dish at Abac packs a surprise. I think chef Jordi Cruz, however, went a bit overboard on the surprise element, as the desire to give customers the unexpected got in the way of taste. Because of that, it's not at the top of my personal list. Abac, where all the meals are a theater in itself, is located in a hotel a little outside of the city. Its wine menu, meanwhile, is very broad at a reasonable cost. I might not be that impressed by the dishes, but the theater of it all is worth a look.

TAPAS 24

Tapas 24 is a tapas bar owned by another chef from the Ferran Adria school, Carles Abellan. Unlike a lot of places on the list, it opens at 9 a.m. and closes at midnight, meaning you can even have breakfast at Tapas 24 (something I certainly enjoy). With a different menu every hour, Tapas 24 allows you to taste crazy dishes that you wouldn't normally find at a traditional tapas bar, like black Russian caviar with fresh avocado or black Spanish truffle eggs. All these interesting combinations are prepared with the tapas spirit. The biggest plus is that there are places to sit outdoors – where it's a good idea to eat outdoors under the shadow of an umbrella protecting you from the hot Barcelona sun... If you want to eat indoors, you have to go down a couple of stairs to the bar.

BERLIN

Everyone knows that Berlin is a city with a huge Turkish population and great Turkish restaurants. I was lucky enough to explore the city with a Berliner and got a chance to sit down for a meal or two in some very interesting restaurants. And thanks to my Berliner guide, I got a peak at the places frequented by the German capital's high society.

The city boasts many famous Turkish restaurants – some of which have done much to make Turkish fare a popular one among Europeans. There are plenty of places with great-tasting food, making the city really lucky in this regard. Berlin might be a big city, but it's eminently walkable or bikable – something to keep in mind when you need to burn off some calories after eating just a bit too much. Below is a list of some of my favorite restaurants in the city, organized, as always, in alphabetical order. The list is according to my own personal taste, but if you go to Berlin and explore new places, please do drop me a line.

ADNAN

Managed by a Berlin-based Turk, Adnan is one of the best restaurants in the city. Although the restaurant is not in a good location, you'll be glad you went, because Adnan's Italian fare is delectable. The place serves almost all the Italian specialties, including pizza, macaroni, salad, meat and fish. Adnan is full at lunch, and the bar is even crowded at dinner. There's a bonus as well: You can find both white and black truffles when they're in season. And for those of you who know that you can get by in Berlin solely speaking Turkish, you won't be surprised to hear that you can order in the language at Adnan.

BORCHARDT

Borchardt is a restaurant that mostly specializes in fish but also serves meat. A favorite of Berlin's high society, Borchardt is a place in which tables are at a premium. As a solution, they hit upon the slightly strange rule of requiring all diners to leave within two hours of arrival. That means that if you got there at 7 p.m., you have to be out by 9 p.m. Or if you start eating at 9 p.m., you have to be on your way by 11. It is, in my opinion, an inconvenient rule, but if you want to experience all that Berlin has to offer, you might just have to accept such rules and regulations. Borchardt does not take great consideration about its décor – it looks like the walls have not been painted for years and it seems like the furnishings haven't been renovated in a coon's age – but it doesn't seem to be a problem for them. On the contrary, Berliners consider this a specialty: You can run a restaurant for 20 or 30 years without doing any renovations – they just reckon that a place's value increases as it gets older.

FISCHERS FRITZ

A fish restaurant with two Michelin stars located inside the Regent Hotel, Fischers Fritz serves dinner (fish and vegetables only) in a comfortable and high-ceilinged space in the company of nice piano music. All the serving staff, as well as the piano player, are women – something that makes for better serving, in my opinion. You needn't worry about finding a place for either lunch or dinner, however, because the restaurant is fairly expensive, in contrast to most eateries in Berlin. Fischers Fritz will especially lighten your wallet, but it is one remarkable restaurant. The restaurant also has a separate entrance from the hotel.

THE GRAND

I have been to Berlin many times before, but I only discovered the Grand thanks to my Berliner guide. The Grand is a meat-heavy restaurant, but it also serves fish and salads. The restaurant serves Japanese Kobe steak, as well as other carnivores' favorites from around the world. A favorite stomping ground of high society, the Grand is another restaurant with its own rules. The Grand is largely off the tourist trail, but that doesn't mean it's not packed with Berliners – all of which means it's a good idea to make reservations ahead of time.

GRILL ROYAL

As its names suggests, Grill Royal is a restaurant that really caters to meat lovers, although you can also find one or two kinds of fish on the menu. Grill Royal is also a fancy restaurant that requires reservations.

KADEWE

Kaufaus des Westens, better known as KaDeWe, is a famous department store in Berlin, and a wonderful place to have a quick and delectable meal. The upper floors of this multistoried mall are reserved for shopping and food, where you can dine at small restaurants on almost any kind of food from anywhere in the world. The very top floor, meanwhile, is home to a big restaurant with an open buffet and mesmerizing views of the city. It's probably my second favourite place in all of Berlin.

I generally opt for oysters, prawns, caviar and lobster – all prepared right in front of you – with the company of a glass of Dom Perignon. After all of that, you'll probably need a good walk to lose those calories, but it's totally worth it!

BOLOGNA

A COUPLE OF DAYS IN THE RED CITY

I've been to the city famous for its rain a number of times, but each time, I was on my way somewhere else. One trip, I finally got the chance to give Bologna my full, undivided attention. Lo and behold, it has some great restaurants that you'd do well to look up if you're ever in the neighborhood.

Until now, I've always visited Bologna while transferring to Florence because there are no direct flights to the famous Tuscan city. (Bologna is just 90 minutes by car from Florence, while its train station, located very close to the local airport, offers good connections to Modena and Venice.) Indeed, I had traveled through Bologna to Modena to dine at Osteria Francescana, one of the world's 50 best restaurants. The brief sojourn in Bologna left an impression, and I always thought that I might return to the city someday. Now I have finally visited the city – and I must say I was pleased with my trip.

For these kinds of short trips, however, I would recommend steering clear of one strong meal after another. If I eat a nice, big meal for lunch, then I generally opt for a light dinner – it's just something that's good for health. More than that, I believe that eating big meals in quick succession takes away from the pleasure you get out of a meal. But while you're making your dinner plans, keep in mind that most restaurants are closed on Sunday evenings!

YOU CAN WALK FOR MILES

They call Bologna "The Red City" because most of the city's buildings are made from red brick. One of the things that left the biggest impression on me was the fact that almost all of the city's buildings have arcades. With so much rain, these arcades – which were mandated by the city authorities long ago on account of the continual deluge from the sky – help you walk for miles without getting a single drop on your head, meaning your sightseeing or shopping can proceed uninterrupted. The arcades are four or five meters wide, providing a great canopy for the pedestrian zone below. (Around 85 percent of the buildings in central Bologna have these arcades, although the newer ones are not as nice as the old ones.)

The arcaded pedestrian ways run for about 12 kilometers, six kilometers of which is closed to vehicle traffic. That means you'll only get wet if you want to cross the road.

For now, it's on to the restaurants! As always, drop me a line with any comments or recommendations of your own.

FIRST STOP: I PORTICI

The hotel I'm recommending in Bologna is I Portici, whose restaurant I also appreciated. I Portici, which has around 40 rooms, is located in an area that is open to vehicular traffic – being able to park right in front of the hotel's door naturally saves you from the trouble of dragging your suitcase down a long road.

The former owner of the building loved music so much so that he built a concert salon for 300-400 people that is topped off with a high ceiling. Today, the old concert salon is used as a restaurant, but that doesn't mean that music has stopped, as there is a piano on the stage where musicians perform every day. I like rooms with high ceilings, so the 8-meter-high ceilings – complete with beautiful frescoes – in the restaurant were positively dazzling.

And one last note: The restaurant at I Portici has a Michelin star.

RISTORANTE BITONE ENOTECA

Ristorante Bitone Enoteca is owned by Cesare, who is like a youngster even in his 70s. He's still cooking and has put together an amazing menu. Everything is perfect, from the wine list to the truffle menu. When I went to dine, they had a truffle the size of a fist (that's not to say that they taste any different than small truffles, although ones as big as this are difficult to find).

Restaurants usually opt to serve small truffles since they are more economic, but chef Cesare spares no expense, choosing instead to use big truffles, which, when trimmed, add to the beauty and visual pleasure of the meal. After all, the presentation of a dish is as important as its taste. Interestingly enough, though, the size of the truffles didn't inflate the bill at all.

We went there as two people and ordered pasta with four kinds of truffle, hoping to try each and every one that had the precious fungus. Chef Cesare, however, had another recipe in mind that we just couldn't keep ourselves from ordering. That's why, in the end, we shared five different pasta dishes with truffle.

AL CAMBIO

Al Cambio is located 15 minutes from the city center. Boasting a Michelin star, Al Cambio is a restaurant with a gastronomic menu that you just have to try. The menu consists of seven or eight courses, all of which are wonderful. The list features both meat and fish; I chose the latter and liked it a lot. Meanwhile, I brought my own wine to the restaurant, thinking I wouldn't be able to find any good wine – not only did they allow me to do this, but they didn't even add any extra charges. As it is, I hardly needed to: Al Cambio has an incredible wine menu, and when I went there, the prices were not even that high.

A BONUS RESTAURANT

RECOMMENDATION: RISTORANTE DIANA

Ristorante Diana is a local little restaurant, 500 meters away from I Portici. I especially recommend its eggs with truffle. If you're planning to just grab a light meal, look no further than Ristorante Diana for something good to eat.

TRUFFLES

The best time to visit Bologna is in October or November, when truffles – particularly white truffles – can be found in the nearby town of Alba... That might bring in a lot of tourists, but it also means that you can sample truffles to your heart's content. Ask your waiter to serve the truffles separately alongside your dish so that you can shave it yourself. That way, you'll be able to breathe in the scent more and experience the whole ceremony of truffles.

CAPE TOWN

Every time I visit Cape Town, I fall in love with it one more time. First of all, the city is home to wonderful restaurants in which you can taste some delectable dishes. Second, its residents have a sincere and natural kindness. The streets are wide but they're not lined with buildings that crowd you out; instead, the city has a very pleasing architectural texture. Unlike Istanbul's coastline, the seaside hasn't been turned into a pile of mortar. From now on, I'll be in Cape Town come February for my summer holiday – you can tag along, too.

I've visited Cape Town twice before. The first was 15 years ago – a time when I was quite interested in golf. I had a wonderful vacation, during which I played on 12 wonderful courses over 12 days in South Africa. It was a very hot summer, but I coped with the weather by playing golf until noon before retiring for a swim in the pool or the sea come afternoon. My second visit to Cape Town was for the World Cup in 2010. During that visit, I watched some of the games played around South Africa, but if the event were to take place again today, I'd only watch the ones played in Cape Town because it's become my favorite and I've fallen in love with it!

With these pleasant thoughts in mind, I had the opportunity to visit Cape Town twice in a row during one winter (for the Northern Hemisphere). The first trip, a four-day visit, was just for business, but the second one in February was for a whole week and, more importantly, just for me! It was an opportunity for me to not only enjoy the city I admired but also revitalize my love for it. And I decided that from now on, if all goes well, I'd visit Cape Town every February. It's the best time of summer there. But for a summer town to appeal to me, it has to have zero humidity, and Cape Town fits the bill, even though it is on the coast. Moreover, it's very affordable. You can have a very nice dinner for half the price you'd pay in some good restaurants in Istanbul.

Today, I want to talk about some of the restaurants I had the pleasure of visiting, as well as a few different vacation itineraries in Cape Town. I'm sure your memories are laden with nice itineraries, beguiling culinary spots and experiences. I'd very much like you to share these – and do let me know if you discover anything new. If you have the chance to visit the places I recommend, let me know what you think at the usual address.

THE WINE WILL DO

I don't think South African wines are really something to write home about, but if you're fine with "not bad," they're pretty affordable. Maybe that's because I'm very demanding when it comes to wine. They're better than the ones in Istanbul but not up to the same standard of those in Bordeaux. Since it has a warm climate, Cape Town has a good harvest of grapes for things like Chardonnay and Riesling – hence, the city's success in producing white wine.

I mentioned that Cape Town is home to nice dishes and restaurants. For me, it has one of the five best restaurants in the world, Test Kitchen – a place that's not on the Michelin list, but that's only because Michelin hasn't entered the market there yet. It's a place, though, that deserves three stars, and you could really journey all the way to Cape Town just for this restaurant.

TEST KITCHEN

Almost half of the restaurant is a kitchen – there's just a counter that divides this large place in two. On one side, they host guests, while on the other, they're cooking the dishes. Equipped with an open kitchen, Test Kitchen resembles a laboratory. The cooks put the meals they've prepared on the counter, the waiters take the dishes and serve them – it's very simple and intimate. It's a relaxing place that's decorated with very nice objects, while it also has a very rich wine menu. You can find beautiful wines from other countries, as well as the best examples of South African wine. If you like, you can take your own wine with you. Whatever the case, you should come prepared for a big meal; it takes three hours in the afternoon and four in the evening (but as someone who's tried both, let me note that the evening menu is preferable). Test Kitchen opens its doors at 7 p.m. for dinner and continues all the way to 11 p.m. It's a long dinner that calls for an empty stomach, so I suggest you skip lunch. It's the only way you can enjoy this 11-course dinner. If you're a vegetarian or prefer fish/meat, you can let them know in advance so that they can organize their menu in accordance with your preferences. (I, for one, really enjoyed the vegetable and fish menu.) Test Kitchen has adapted a fusion-dominant culinary approach in which they use fruit in a number of dishes – I especially liked their sweet-and-sour sauce that was made from fruit.

And a few bits and bobs: They like to serve their fish and seafood undercooked... The last three courses are cheese, dessert and fruit. And one more word to the wise: The visual presentation of the dishes is great, but it's even better if you watch the cooks prepare and the waiters serve these delicious dishes.

HARBOUR HOUSE

Harbour House is a lot like the fish restaurants by the sea in Istanbul. There's no fixed menu; they just have a few large blackboards on which they write the day's dishes and prices. When you arrive, a couple of waiters bring one of these boards to your table; you examine the board, consult the waiter and make a pick. But what's really best is this: The waiter lets you know which fish on the menu is fresh and which one was frozen the day before because it went unsold. This information isn't written on the board, but you can get up to speed while giving your order. Harbour House has developed a special way to define the difference between the two: that day's fish is called "fresh," while the frozen ones are called "freshly frozen." As it's an open sea right in front of you, the fish is great, and the local abundance of crawfish, spring lobster, lobster and shrimp is reflected on the menu. My favorite, though, was the grilled fish – while the big bowl of salad they also serve makes this place an ideal restaurant for me. In terms of a drink, you can enjoy your meal with a selection of South African wines.

Located in Waterfront (a very popular district in Cape Town), Harbour House also has a branch in Kalk Bay. Some 45 minutes away from Cape of Good Hope, Kalk Bay is situated right after the Cape of

Good Hope – the place where the Atlantic Ocean ends and the Indian Ocean begins. Sparing a thought for visitors who might want to take a dip in the water, the restaurant built concrete walls in the sea to serve as a pool. Holes in the walls at the water line also enable the water to circulate. And those worried about their swimming skills need not worry inordinately, as there are lifeguards on duty.

NOBU

The most prominent restaurant in Cape Town is Nobu, an accessible place with very high ceilings by the seaside, as well as a fantastic outdoor eating area. The wine menu, which also includes the most famous of South African wines, is more than satisfactory. The dishes, seating plan and ambiance is also brilliant. My favorite here is the cod; dubbed Black Cod on the menu, this dish is wrapped in a leaf and served in a mildly sweet sauce.

The hotel bar next door is transformed into a hip place on Saturday evenings; boasting a spectacular view, the place can serve a thousand people. My advice to you is to enjoy a few aperitifs and a pleasant conversation at the hotel bar before decamping downstairs to Nobu for the feast of your life.

AN UTTERLY DIFFERENT EXPERIENCE: GRAFF

Now, let me turn my attention to a couple of places that double up as both hotels and restaurants in the Paarl and Stellenbosch districts, which are home to many wineries. Forty-five minutes outside of town, Paarl and Stellenbosch are close enough for a day trip, although they are home to two wonderful hotels. The first one is Graff. Opened by a famous Dutch diamond merchant, Graff is a well-known winery and hotel. The wines meet South African standards, but the restaurant and hotel are out of this world. It's just a boutique, 10-room hotel (five of which overlook a cliff with vineyards), but don't let the small size fool you – each room boasts close to 200 square meters, and each room possesses a garden of equal size. Even better, each garden has an outdoor swimming pool that's solely for the use of the room's occupant. And there are no worries about privacy, as tall trees surrounding the pool and garden prevent any outside intrusion.

Open up your sliding door and it's as if the room becomes one with the garden. What's more, the pool is a mere two steps from your bed in the morning. Everything's designed to provide maximum comfort and pleasure to guests. After checking in, a member of the hotel staff knocks on your door, carrying a big tray. He leaves a bottle of champagne in an ice bucket, as well as a fruit basket on the table, and inquires as to when he can come later. He then comes at the appointed hour, this time with a bottle of white wine in ice, canapes and snacks.

Graff also has a wonderful restaurant, but you have to make a reservation a month in advance. It has an à la carte menu featuring an array of international cuisine. It's a beautiful place overlooking kilometers of vineyards. They have a menu of wines, most of which are homemade. Of course, the most appealing aspect of this place is the personal luxury and atmosphere they provide.

For the hotel, you need to make a reservation

three months in advance. I had duly made my reservation well in advance for the restaurant but didn't think the same amount of forethought was necessary for the hotel. Needless to say, I couldn't find a room. But a friend of mine, who knows the hotel owner – the jewelry merchant Graff – came to the rescue. I could only stay one night, but it was, as you would expect, a wonderful experience.

BABYLONSTOREN

Housing 20 large rooms and a restaurant, Babylonstoren is another of my favorites. Graff is rich in luxury, while Babylonstoren is rich in plainness – it's almost like a campsite. They place so much emphasis on ecological balance that they don't even put chlorine in the hotel's pool. Plain though it may be, Babylonstoren is popular, and you need to make a reservation for the hotel and restaurant at least one month in advance. Its biggest merit is the fact that the ingredients used in the food, including the meat, are organic and raised or cultivated on farms nearby. The only thing that they source from outside is the daily fish.

RECOMMENDATIONS...

RENT A HOUSE IF YOU'RE STAYING A WHILE

Cape Town's five-star hotels cost as much as their counterparts in Europe, but it's possible to find three- or four-star hotels that are quite affordable. However, if you're planning to stay for a month, you can rent a house for 400-500 euros per month in a luxurious district.

A COMFORTABLE TRIP

If you're coming from Turkey, Turkish Airlines operates nightly flights to Cape Town. The flight departs at 1 a.m. and lands in the morning. It takes 12-13 hours, but it's a very comfortable trip if you can manage to get some sleep. But despite the long duration, there's obviously no jetlag if you're coming from Turkey or elsewhere in Europe. The return flight, meanwhile, is at 4 p.m.

FOR GOLF ENTHUSIASTS

I'd like to add one more restaurant, especially for golf enthusiasts: Catherina's at Steenberg. Serving a menu that focuses on fish, the restaurant is located on a golf course 20 minutes from town. If you like playing golf and care about what you eat, it's definitely worth a try.

CATALONIA

For five years, I had done everything in my power to try and go to El Bulli, a restaurant without rival. I even solicited the assistance of some Spanish acquaintances, all to no avail. But after a long struggle, I finally found the opportunity to dine at El Bulli thank to the efforts of a close friend. For that, I am most grateful.

El Bulli closed its doors a number of years ago, and it will remain shut for some time to come. During this long hiatus, its chef will take a rest, the restaurant will redevelop its menu and workers will renovate the place. Twenty days before El Bulli closed, however, I got a chance to go and experience their spectacular menu. Without exaggeration, I can say it is the most delicious meal I ever had – not just because of the taste but also because of its general quality, the dishes, the service and the drinks. There's no El Bulli to go to right now, but even if there were, they would be taking reservations a year in advance.

Given such an enjoyable culinary experience, El Bulli deserves almost a full article all by itself. When it was open, El Bulli was typically open from April to October. Diners could never avail themselves of an à la carte menu; instead the meal consisted of a fixed menu of 25 to 45 small plates (the menu would only change once a year) spread over five hours (after all, how would you get through so many dishes any quicker?). The chef, the 50-year-old Ferran Adria, has been cooking since he was a child, and when El Bulli was open, his kitchen was as big as the adjoining 50-person restaurant. Employed in the kitchen were 50 cooks, putting the cook-guest ratio at 1:1.

EL BULLI IN THE ART EXHIBITION

Too many cooks in the kitchen didn't spoil the broth, but instead made El Bulli's food into an art form – so much so that the curators of the DOCUMENTA Art Exhibition asked Ferran to lend his culinary creations to their event, which was held in 2007 in Kassel, Germany. Ferran agreed, but he also noted that he wouldn't be able to show off his creations in Germany because his food required local ingredients if it was going to be good. Accordingly, Ferran suggested to the curators that they bring the exhibition to his restaurant so that visitors could come and see the installation there. In fact, he even gave two lucky visitors a chance to dine in his restaurant every day. Ultimately, the DOCUMENTA event allowed 200 people to dine at El Bulli over the 100 days of the biennial.

Over the years, I've read several books about Ferran in an effort to learn what makes him tick. Like him, the restaurant also has an original story. In 1961, a German doctor, Hans Schilling, and his wife, Marketta, came to the small town of Roses, which is northeast of Barcelona near the French border. Long before the area became popular, they bought land at a low price on the shore of a small and shimmering cove before proceeding to build a summer house. Later, they decided to enlarge the house to turn it into a fast-food restaurant to serve the many beachgoers who came to the area.

In time, the restaurant grew, even if the Schillings' love did not; they divorced, although their restaurant partnership continued, as Hans brought materials and equipment to develop their business.

Soon, they hired a French chef to take their restaurant to the next level before renaming the establishment "El Bulli," the Spanish words for bulldog, in honor of their own dog of the same breed.

The restaurant won its first star as a French restaurant in 1976, eight years before Ferran arrived on the scene as an assistant chef. In time, the boss left to start his own business, leaving Ferran in charge. El Bulli obtained its second star in 1990 and a third in 1997.

Meanwhile, the restaurant was managed by Julie Soler, who was looking after the marketing, supervision of staff and reservations, while Ferran's brother, Albert, had begun working as the pastry chef. As the years progressed, the original owners sold the restaurant to Julie and Ferran, who chose to keep the restaurant closed over the winter to turn their attention to new recipes. The closure – as well as the quest for new recipes – soon became a tradition.

YEARS AT THE PINNACLE

Every year, the world's best chefs vote for the planet's best restaurant, and for four years (from 2006 to 2009), El Bulli was selected the best restaurant in the world (it also finished second in 2010). Needless to say, El Bulli has an excellent reputation among chefs.

During El Bulli's run, nearly 8,000 people dined there every year. At the start of a new year, customers would seek to make reservations, but there was no guarantee that you would find a spot during the calendar year. If you had happened to dine there before, however, then you might be in luck, since half of the 8,000-person capacity was reserved for regular customers. For those who hadn't dined there before, they had to ride their luck and hope to be one of the 4,000 out of the 2 million – yes, 2 million – to win a reservation at the restaurant. After winning a place, lucky customers would pay for the meal in advance by credit card. (But pity those who won a reservation for a date they could not attend; instead of getting a second pick of date, El Bulli would cancel their reservation and select another person from the hundreds of thousands of prospective diners.) In this way, the restaurant met its expenses for its yearly April opening by the beginning of January.

With such demand, El Bulli's managers could have easily capitalized on the place's reputation and opened brunches in different cities of the world. They could also have opened the place at noon or kept the restaurant open the whole year, thereby doubling their income. The thing is, they didn't want to: Ferran Adria is an artistic person, and he preferred to take some rest instead of working hard.

As for me, I spent five years, fruitlessly sending emails in the hopes of becoming one of the 4,000 selected to dine at El Bulli. But thanks to the intervention of a friend, I finally got to join that select club.

A 42-PORTION EXTRAVAGANZA
The menu would consist of 42 servings that would come every seven minutes. El Bulli would also serve very nice wine with the food – which is one of the reasons I was happy that we traveled by taxi, as it allowed me to partake more than if I had taken my

own car. As you might expect, however, a meal there was expensive.

Tasting the menu was an interesting experience, as just 12 of the 42 servings were geared to our palette, while the rest of them were surprising in every way! At one point, for instance, they served something that looked just like a big, white, Easter egg; we dug in, expecting it to be chocolate, only to find that it was nothing but cheese! The dish, which tasted like parmesan, melted in the mouth immediately. As we clamored about to try more of it, we suddenly realized that we had finished it all.

After the "Easter egg," we were served what we thought was caviar – only to have something that tasted like hazelnut. El Bulli would make a lot of surprises like these during your special dinner.

Ultimately a humble man, Ferran showed us around the restaurant, gave us a book as a gift and even engaged in some small take despite not being so proficient in English.

ANOTHER CATALAN STAR: CAN ROCA

The other restaurant with three Michelin stars in Catalonia is the El Celler de Can Roca. The restaurant, which was selected the second best in the world this year, is in Girona, which is about 90 minutes from Barcelona. Three brothers own the place: Joan Roca (executive chef), Joseph Roca (sommelier) and Jordi Roca (pastry chef).

The restaurant, which has a capacity for about 60 or 70 people, is in a very nice and modern building. They have an option for an à la carte menu, but I would suggest trying the 12-portion menu, which is accompanied by very suitable and affordable wine. The place impressed me so much that I will definitely visit there again. It might not be El Bulli, but Can Roca still throws up some nice surprises!

In the end, I would recommend the lunch at Can Roca. Although the menu "only" has 11 or 12 servings (a far cry from El Bulli's 42), it also takes upwards of five hours to eat.

THE CLOSEST STAR TO BARCELONA: CAN FABES

Can Fabes is a restaurant with three Michelin stars about 45 minutes out of Barcelona (it acquired its last star in 1994). There is also a mini hotel on site, meaning you can dine and spend the night there as well.

All of these restaurants are remarkable, but if I would have to rank them, I would put Can Fabes in third place – which, given how successful a restaurant it is, just goes to show how challenging the Catalan competition is.

Although Can Fabes is more of a standard place, it does have a six- or seven-portion menu, although its wine selection is fairly ordinary. You can have an appetizer, a main course and a dessert.

Can Fabes also has a Spanish chef who is on bad terms with El Bulli. The chef frequently criticizes Ferran Adria's work, declaring himself someone who cooks real food – unlike Ferran Adria's "artificial meals."

THE CHALLENGE OF BEING AN INTERN AT EL BULLI

While it was open, El Bulli used to receive about 2,500 applications per year from chefs who wanted to become unpaid interns at the famous restaurant. These interns, mind you, were no kids right out of high school, but 30-somethings who were already up to great things, like being the owners or executive chefs of a restaurant. Only 20 to 50 of these 2,500 were selected to intern at El Bulli, where they had the opportunity to learn in the presence of Ferran Adria.

Receiving just room and board for 12 months, the interns would work on El Bulli's next menu for when the restaurant would reopen after winter. Some popular dishes tended to reappear in the new menus, but many of the rest were entirely new!

COPENHAGEN

This time, I happened to find myself in a realm far away, Copenhagen. The city might be cold and northern, but I discovered an amazing place and extraordinary dishes. Let me share a bit about my time in the Danish capital. And if you go, will you like Noma as much as I did?

So, what's so special about this restaurant that sits a mere 40 at lunch and 40 for dinner? However did this Copenhagen restaurant, which has been named top restaurant three times in a row, come out on top in a city where the sun, farming and food diversity are below average? What's more, the restaurant is located in an average neighborhood without any special view. (It might be near the seaside, but a lot of things in Copenhagen are, so that's not a stunning feat.)

WHAT'S THE SECRET?

Noma's chef, the fortyish Rene Redzepi, was born and raised in Copenhagen but is the child of a Macedonian family. He mainly cooks fish and vegetables, but he is also a stickler for using fresh food who really cares about using seasonal harvest. Accordingly, Rene offers a constantly changing, if also narrow, menu.

Rene gets most of his ingredients from Denmark, only procuring some of his fish from further afield like Greenland, Iceland and the islands of South America.

Noma still has just two Michelin stars, but it perhaps deserves a third given how much it's finishing first in competitions. Located in a former store room in a stone building that was converted into its current form, Noma boasts high ceilings and a fair degree of comfort.

I had long wished to visit Noma, but constantly failed to find a chance to book. But thanks again to the intervention of my friend Mehmet Gürs, I was able to make a reservation for a Saturday night. And let me tell you, I couldn't be happier.

If you accompany your meal with alcohol, you might have to part with 200 euros for the whole affair. It might seem pricy, but considering how popular the Michelin-approved restaurant is, the prices are actually quite reasonable.

A TRUE SUCCESS STORY

Rene left school at the age of 15 and started studying culinary arts at a simple institution. After graduating, he began working in restaurants as a busboy. At the age of 20, he found work as a chef at a nice restaurant in France. After that, he made his way further south, heading to El Bulli, where he stayed for a couple of years and learned all one can about the ins and outs of the legendary Catalan restaurant. Looking for something knew, he headed stateside for a new experience, succeeding in finding a job at Napa Valley's The French Laundry, a world-famous establishment owned by Thomas Keller, who also owns Per Se. After working at The French Laundry for a while, he decided to return home to Denmark, where he converted an empty warehouse into a restaurant. In time, Rene started to show off his skills, earning himself a global reputation.

Today, you have scant chance of booking a table at Noma through any ordinary channels. Perhaps you might be able to score a reservation through the intervention of someone you know, although there is another – albeit slightly riskier – option available to you: Go to the restaurant's bar at about 7 p.m.; after spending some time there, insist on some food and, if the stars align, you might just succeed. This course of action, however, is probably only wise for a single person – I certainly wouldn't recommend it if you are two or more people. Luckily, I didn't have to try my chances with this method as Mehmet Gürs was on hand to help. I am eminently grateful for his assistance.

DIFFERENT COOKS FOR DIFFERENT DISHES

Noma has a gastronomical menu that includes nine main courses cooked by different cooks. In the Noma system, chef groups of three or four people cook and serve the same meal – generally easily prepared meals – for a whole day. For each dish, the head of the group of chefs comes to your table to introduce the meal. (That is why you constantly see chefs walking around the restaurant's dining section.)

Rene mostly uses oil olive for the meals. He also uses plenty of vegetables and herbs for an intensive flavor and smell. He grows these herbs himself in the restaurant's closed section, as it's hard to find all the necessary vegetables come winter (although it might not be that onerous a task in which only 80 people are dining each day). Rene also uses these herbs for the sauce and garniture.

Another important feature at Noma is their use of a technique to dry food by draining it. They mix these dry foods with others or, alternatively, make them crispy before serving. In this way, they turn porcini mushrooms, sea scallops and carrots into something resembling chips. The Scandinavians often smoke their food, such as salmon, to preserve it. Rene, naturally, uses this method as well, and it is possible to find all manners of smoked meat, fish and vegetables on the menu.

A SPECTACULAR WINE MENU

Noma has an extraordinary wine menu. Whenever I go to a place, I'm generally familiar with about half the names on the wine menu because of my special interest of wine. At Noma, however, I was at a loss: I didn't know almost 90 percent of the wines on the restaurant's   menu.

As I learned later, Noma's sommelier provides small amounts of wine that it sources from small brands, bringing wines that are produced in Denmark, Germany and Holland in limited runs. I let the sommelier select the wines for me, as I wanted to taste different wines instead of drinking a whole bottle. The sommelier started me off with a white Chardonnay from Denmark. Now a Chardonnay is a kind of grape that generally prefers hot climes, but I enjoyed this natural and non-barrelled wine. When I asked for a second glass, however, they told me that they had run out of the white Chardonnay, offering me a white Sauvignon Blanc from Copenhagen instead.

After that, they offered me a glass of an Italian wine made in 2004. I love it – in fact, I drank a couple glasses of it. I liked the wine so much that I noted down the name, later getting in contact with the producer. As luck would have it, though, they had already sold all of their product from 2004; I didn't want to waste my money on the vintage of another year, so I abandoned the quest.

Now, Noma serves wine in small drinking cups – something I generally cannot abide since most places typically serve cheap and tasteless win in such vessels. At Noma, however, the experience was more than fine, as I got to sample plenty of top-quality wines at the same time.

AN APPEALING VISUALITY

Depending on the workload, there are about 40-50 people who work at the restaurant, 30 of whom are cooks. They're all young people in casual outfits – you won't see any waiter in a black tie.

Copenhagen is a city in which you rarely see the color green, but Noma compensates for the lack of green with its dishes that are grown in the kitchen. Meanwhile, they make use of herbs by draining them to color up the dishes. Ultimately, Rene cooks delicious meals with fresh fish and spices in a city where vegetables and other ingredients are restricted.

I and the other 2,000 people that have come to eat Rene's creations over the past three years are of the same opinion: Noma is a remarkable restaurant. They can serve 40 people at a time at Noma; they could expand the restaurant's capacity if they wanted, but they don't, even though 4,000 people try and make reservations for Noma every year. I appreciate the restaurant's policy of insisting on the quality of the food instead of earning more money. The same goes for any successful chef and their restaurants. I can't wait to taste Noma's delicious food again.

FLORENCE

FLORENCE, THE HEART OF THE RENAISSANCE

Without question, Florence is the most important city in Tuscany, but more than that, it is a city of unparalleled significance in both Italy and Europe. The spiritual home of the renaissance, it also has plenty of restaurants, winehouses and hotels. Today, let me tell you about just a few of my favorites.

But beyond that, let me tell you about a few places that you must see. Now, there are more than a few tour guides in Florence who can tell you where to go if you haven't been there before, but how many of them can tell you where to go if you've been there several times before?

WAKE UP IN A PALACE

My favorite hotel in Florence is the Four Seasons. Around 150 years ago, the building was the mansion of a rich Florentine, but has since been renovated and converted into a hotel, frescoes and all. In fact, they did such a good job that Four Seasons now considers the hotel to be the best of its brand in Europe.

That it most certainly is. It's true, we do have a couple of Four Seasons in Turkey, and they're pretty good, but the Four Seasons in Florence is something else. The hotel boasts a 15th-century garden that stretches for over an acre – something that is welcome in a crowded city like Florence. And if you stay in one of the luxury rooms, you can't help but feel like an Italian aristocrat. My recommendation to you is to stay in the hotel's "Gallery Suit," which is bedecked in frescoes that cover the walls and ceiling. The room has a view of the Giardino Gherardesca, an expanse of green that is sure to impress you in the same way that the Bosphorus takes away the breath of any Istanbulite. There's even an enormous tree in the center of the garden in which 30 people could easily stand underneath and be hidden from view.

The hotel also has a fantastic restaurant called Il Palagio, which is headed by the extremely talented chef Vito. The restaurant, which has two separate sections for both summer and winter, serves delicious dishes at every meal, including brunch. And although the wine cellar is spectacular, it won't take a bite out of your wallet. Instead, you pay only about two times the bulk price – a far cry from the three or four times the bulk price that you usually pay at a fancy place like this. And better than that, you need not be a hotel guest to dine at Il Palagio. Still, given the garden, restaurant, wine cellar (and spa), you wouldn't go wrong in staying here for night.

Like Istanbul's Çırağan Palace, the Four Seasons has another modern building in its garden that is separate from the historical main building. If you're looking for a cheaper stay, this is the place for you.

Paul, who is the most talented concierge I have ever seen, can manage everything for you. If you stay at the Four Seasons, I strongly recommend you go straight to Paul and surrender yourself to his skills. A fixer who knows everybody in town, Paul can immediately step in whenever you want to book a place for an event.

THE BEST TWO RESTAURANTS IN FLORENCE

Enoteca Pinchiorri is not only the best restaurant in Florence, it's also the best in Italy. A three-star affair, the Pinchiorri is an extremely elegant place and, if I may say so myself, a little bit on the snobby side. A simple, three-course meal will run you 150 euros – and that's without any wine. If you do want to imbibe, that will set you back a whopping 500 euros per person. Leaving this aside, the place, wine, food and service are remarkable.

My second suggestion in Florence is Cibreo, a family business where the prices are more down to earth. There are, in fact, two Cibreos in Florence, both of which belong to the same family. One is more in the style of a café, with wooden tables and no reservations required. The other – the one I will recommend (while acknowledging that the first Cibreo is a good place for a spot of lunch if you're planning to stay in Florence for a while) – requires reservations and boasts a well-functioning service.

You'll soon realize that Cibreo serves up a different taste when you see that there's no pasta on the menu – a seemingly massive oversight given that you're in Italy! More than that, there are also no rib roasts, another popular meal in the country.

OTHER RESTAURANTS

Florence may be far from the sea, but you can still find fresh, daily fish in the restaurant Fuor d'Acqua, where the menu has nothing but things from the sea. The restaurant also offers a bit of a tavern atmosphere. Though Fuor d'Acqua's service isn't perfect, its appetizers and fish are impeccable. The place is similar to our Urcan Restaurant of yesteryear. If you've got four or five days in Florence, then it's a place that is worth a meal.

FANTASTIC ITALIAN WINES

Leave aside the restaurants for now and come with me to a couple of winehouses. One belongs to the Antinori family, the biggest wine producer in Italy. Even today, the third generation of the family still produces wine – although the members of this generation are estranged from each other to the point that they have become rivals. Regardless, the family members who have preserved the name Antinori have wineries in both Italy and overseas. In the environs of Florence, the closest is in the Badia region, a place about 20 minutes away in which Cabarnet Sauvignon and Shiraz grapes are cultivated. Antinori has a small winery here in which you can taste their product, eat some food and find almost every range of wine for purchase. After a bit of breakfast is a great time to arrange a visit to the vineyards, watch the winemakers at work and have a wee taste. The restaurant is also the perfect place to take a break and enjoy a light lunch.

My second suggestion is Castello di Montauto, a 30-minute drive away in the San Gimignano region. What's at the end of the road is wonderful, but the journey itself is worth an after-breakfast trip because the roads and views are mesmerizing. Castello di Montauto is a small and modern winehouse with a wonderful garden that makes an excellent place for a light, noon-day meal.

If you have two mornings in Florence, definitely make an effort to take in these two winehouses.

ART, ARCHITECTURE AND THE MARKET
There are more than a few, must-see places in Florence, but here are five of them!

1. Constructed in 1560, the Galleria degli Uffizi is the most important art gallery in Florence.

2. The Galleria dell'Accademia boasts a treasure trove of artwork from the renaissance.

3. If you want to visit a palace, look no further than the Palazzo Pitti, near the Galleria dell'Accademia.

4. Ponte Vecchio is the oldest and most famous bridge over the Arno River. The link between the two sides of Florence also features plenty of souvenir shops.

5. The Cathedral Santa Maria Del Fiore is a fantastic church with an impressive interior and exterior.

Half a day is enough to visit these five places, as they're not located too far apart from one another. If you have the time, though, take a bit longer to visit them so that you soak in all the ambience.

After all that sight-seeing, I suggest you visit the Santa Croce Square. Sit down, order a coffee and enjoy some people-watching.

WHAT'S THE BEST WAY TO GET THERE?
If you're coming from Turkey, there's no direct flight to Florence. If you absolutely must fly into Florence,

opt for a Lufthansa flight passing through Munich or Frankfurt. If there is a delay, however, you might miss your connecting flight.

Alternatively, Turkish Airlines now operates direct flights to Bologna, from which it's just 90 minutes by car. Another option is to fly to Rome and then make the 2.5-hour drive to the Tuscan jewel. That, however, takes a long time, so I would suggest you go for the Bologna option.

HAVANA

It's no secret that I generally opt to visit cities with some excellent restaurants, but this time, I plumped for something different: Cuba. I spent days immersed in all the dancing and music that Cuba has to offer, joining the locals who somehow manage to live happily despite everything they lack. Just don't ask about the food…

I've been to many places in the world, some even more than once, but I had always put off going to Cuba. Why, you ask? First, it's a faraway place that's really hard to reach with a direct flight. Second, I've always heard that the island's food is nothing to write home about. With beautiful restaurants and good food my main reason to travel, why would I go to Cuba when there are all these other countries and cities with wonderful restaurants? But my resistance to my friends' entreaties finally cracked, and I decided to give it a go. The friends in question – one Italian, one Turkish – have visited Cuba every autumn for the past decade, typically staying there for a few weeks each time. They presented me with such a good itinerary that it was impossible to say "no" this time around. For one, they rented an apartment in the tallest privately owned building in Havana, hired a host that speaks great English and provided a vehicle with a chauffeur.

But before anything else, the most beautiful thing in Cuba is life itself. The people may not be rich, but they sure are happy. You hear wonderful music everywhere. Everybody's either dancing or making music. Havana also boasts a pedestrianized street –

one that's much like Istanbul's İstiklal Avenue – that runs for about two kilometers. The street is lined with numerous cafés and bars, all of which emit all manners of music – yet thankfully not to the degree that it drowns out the music of their neighbors. Whether it's a double bass accompanied by a saxophone or a piano and a guitar, everyone makes lovely music.

The historical buildings and natural charm of the city create a whole other atmosphere. It baffles you to see such happy people live such poverty-stricken lives. For instance, I visited a cigar factory where hundreds of people work, yet earn a mere 35 dollars a month. Nevertheless, some of the factory workers were singing while others were keeping the beat.

But if I had 10 meals during my seven-day visit there, I couldn't finish my dish at nine of them, such were the dishes' unappealing nature. If I were to visit Cuba again, it would probably only be for the music and the dancing – that is, for the fun. (Although it might be a great way to lose a few pounds again without pushing myself too hard.)

A TÊTE-À-TÊTE WITH HEMINGWAY

One must-see place at the center of Cuba's nightlife is the famous bar El Floridita. During his years in Havana, Ernest Hemingway would come here and write short stories while sipping a daiquiri. And in homage to the great writer, a bronze statue bearing his likeness now graces what was once his regular seat. El Floridita's walls are covered with Hemingway's photographs, as well as those of Fidel Castro. The bar serves a variety of aperitifs, including at least 20 kinds of daiquiri. Their specialty, however, is the appropriately named Floridita Daiquiri, which has very little sugar in it. During our week in Cuba, El Floridita was a place we made sure to visit every day. Naturally, it also has great music, with the orchestra changing several times a day.

WHERE TO EAT?
While in Cuba, I went to a lot of restaurants, but I can't say I liked any of them except one – La Casa, a restaurant where a blonde cook looking more Swedish than Cuban cooks the dishes. True to its name, La Casa really is a home: It's a family-owned, three-story house, half of which is a living area for the fairly large family, while the other half is used as a restaurant. Cubans have to pay a sum of nearly 40,000 dollars to own a house, so it doesn't take a mathematical whiz to compute that that's a princely sum given that the average wage is just 35 dollars a month.

The family, though, has an ace up their sleeve: They own another house in a fishing village about 20-25 minutes outside Havana. That's a big plus, because the state only sells frozen fish to ensure they don't spoil in the country's hot climate. It's a good move in terms of public health policy, but it's pretty annoying if you want to dig into some fresh fish. The restaurant's cook visits the fishermen early every morning and buys as much as he serve that day (provided the state hasn't yet purchased all the fish) – that's why the menu never specifies what kind of fish it'll be other than inform customers that it'll be "today's fish."

Almost every member of the family works at the restaurant. The elders look after the kids, while the youth work either as waiters or cooks. The cook's aunt, meanwhile, makes the most delicious ice cream I've ever had in my life. The pineapple-flavored concoction is served in, what else, a pineapple while coconut ice cream comes in a coconut. But no matter how hard I tried, I couldn't get her to give me the secret recipe. Still, I have a few ideas as to how she makes it, and I've made up my mind to figure it out through trial and error. I really enjoyed La Casa; if ever I visit Cuba again, that's where I'll eat the whole time.

There's one other restaurant in Havana that I liked: Rio Mare. This place also serves fish but, for the reasons outlined above, they're frozen. They also have great pasta, side dishes and desserts. Rio Mare is situated next to the water, much like the fish restaurants along the Bosphorus. If you're sitting at one of the tables by the window, you can even touch the water. They have a great wine list – offering a surprising mix for Cuban standards. Somehow, the restaurant managed to get imported wines into the country and put them on the menu. You may wish to steer clear of the frozen fish, but you can satiate yourself with fresh lobster (which, in contrast to the fish, is very easy to find), alongside a nice bottle of wine.

WHERE TO STAY?
We stayed at a penthouse in a 25-story building called Atlantic Tower, which overlooks the ocean. The price was affordable enough for us, although it was obviously expensive by Cuban standards. In fact, the place (which also had a pool and a terrace) was so large that it could have comfortably hosted four couples. And when locals heard where we were staying, they all

raised an eyebrow. To put it another way, we became the cool kids on the block thanks to the apartment. But if you're not interested in the penthouse, I can recommend three other hotels for accommodation.

The first is Hotel Nacional – a one-time hospital that is very nice despite its somewhat disorderly appearance. The Nacional, which bears more than a passing resemblance to Istanbul's Pera Palas, is situated among the trees in the middle of Havana. Even if you don't stay there, come by at night to catch one of the live performances. The second hotel is Saratoga. Located in the city center, the place is convenient in that it's within the aforementioned pedestrianized area, meaning you can experience all the vibrancy and color that the street has to offer. I'm not sure about the food at the foreign-owned hotel but I did like the rooms I had the chance to see.

Santa Isabel is another hotel overlooking a central square. It has a terrace that gets the sun from a beautiful angle, especially after noon, making it the perfect spot to have a sandwich and a few drinks by the sea. The Santa Isabel also has high ceilings and well-maintained rooms. The prices are also reasonable, with standard rooms starting at 100 dollars a night and rising to up to 300 dollars.

WHAT TO DRINK?

Beer, daiquiris, piña coladas and, of course, rum are all in abundance in Cuba. No matter where you drink beer – whether at a luxurious hotel or at the market on the corner – the price is just 2 dollars, the standard beer price set by the government. The national Cuban drink, however, is rum. Just don't get your hopes up for the wine, though – it's awful!

In terms of Havana's understanding of entertainment, the fun starts every day at 12 p.m. and continues right on until midnight or later. But even a walk of a few hours during the day may turn into a great visual feast as you encounter acrobats, music bands dressed in carnival costumes and many others... And then, of course, there are the cigar shops, which have become synonymous with the country. In some shops, you can watch how the cigars are made and buy some if you'd like. I don't smoke myself, but a gift of some of Cuba's finest did go well with friends back home who are into cigars.

During my sojourn, I lost almost five pounds because I couldn't eat anything – it was a sort of detox for me. But I had a great time drinking a couple of bottles of beer since I couldn't find any decent wine.

While there, we even threw a party at our apartment. My one friend said he knew a lot of people there and that we'd have great fun if we threw a party. "I'll do the cooking," I said, beginning the preparations. We ended up being 14 people, including a dancing couple who sang and played percussion, Giselle (a famous singer in Havana), our chauffeur, as well as his father, who had a lovely voice. The only Turks at the party were my friend and I. Everyone sang songs accompanied by a guitar and percussion for about two hours. In fact, they have a tradition that's similar to the battle of the poets/musicians in Turkish folk literature: Men and women gather in two different groups and face one another before one side picks a sentence for a made-up melody. The other group forms another sentence that rhymes with the previous and, of course, is accompanied by a made-up rhythm. The side that fails to come up with a rhyme loses – although the ultimate point is to dance, sing and have fun! I, for one, pulled my weight at the party by serving a delicious swordfish to the guests.

TIPS FOR EXPLORATION

If you don't mind parting with too much cash, you can always get about by one of Havana's old classic taxis for about 30 dollars a trip. It takes about 20 minutes to get from one place to another. If you're just traveling about town once or twice – and especially if you want to try out the old classic cars – these taxis are fine, although they're not a good idea if you're journeying beyond Havana, since they break down easily. Alternatively, another option is to hire a chauffeur for about 90 dollars a day. Typically, such drivers operate five- or six-year-old Japanese, Chinese or Korean cars. Ultimately, it's much cheaper and advantageous to hire cars with chauffeurs, particularly ones with a smattering of English (after all, it only takes about 50 words to take care of everything here). You should also carry your credit card and passport at all times, but be advised that they don't accept American Express (probably because of the name). And though they do accept U.S. dollars, paying by credit card is more advantageous due to the exchange rate.

A PLACE YOU NEED TO SEE: CASA DEL MUSICA

Located in the Miramare region, the dance club Casa del Musica only opens its doors at midnight. Here (beyond the music, of course) it really is just about the drinks: They only serve beverages, meaning there are no hors d'oeuvres, no nuts, no carrots, nothing. Come midnight, an orchestra takes the stage and performs until about 3 a.m., providing ample opportunity for everyone to dance the night away. And if you're a non-smoker, you're in luck: There is no smoking indoors – which is part of the reason there's always a congregation of people outside having a puff.

HONG KONG

I was 20 years younger the last time I visited Hong Kong.

The view is absolutely stunning when you gaze at the island from the mainland, but it's not the same when you do it vice versa. Two decades on, I still think the same things about Hong Kong, a place with a vibrant social life. And, in actuality, the passing years have only added a few buildings to the silhouette of the city.

The last time I was here, I stayed at a hotel on the mainland, enjoying a room with a view of the island. With a desire to experience something different, I stayed in Hong Kong proper this time. On our first night on the island, we dined at Lung King Heen – a restaurant with three Michelin stars. The restaurant was a beautiful, à la carte Chinese restaurant with a small testing menu. The wine menu was also wide, yet it wasn't so high in price.

I can easily say that Hong Kong is a place where you can find every wine imaginable – and at very reasonable prices. Almost all restaurants sell wines of high quality at a relatively inexpensive price thanks to tax breaks and high demand. So look no further than the island for a chance to sample the very best of French or American wine.

The specifically Chinese restaurant we went to the next day, Tang Court, was located in the Langham Hotel. Though a restaurant with two Michelin stars, Tang Court has absolutely no windows and, thus, no view. Nevertheless, Tang Court is a pretty good choice for a dinner thanks to its fair prices and Michelin standards. And one top tip: the Tang Court's Peking duck is fantastic…

OZONE BAR

The Ozone Bar is located on the 118th floor of the tallest hotel in the world, the 490-meter Ritz Carlton Hong Kong. Unsurprisingly, the Ozone Bar has a fairly breathtaking view of the island. There are no fancy Michelin stars here, but the place is famous for its kitchen, view and fine drinks. Four or five years have passed since the opening of the bar, but it's stealing customers from the two-Michelin-star restaurant located in the Ritz Carlton. If you prefer a night view, then reserve your place for a dinner, but if you're more of a morning-view person, hit the place for lunch.

If you like fusion cuisine then Hong Kong's Zuma or Roca are the places to dine. The service at both is excellent. If you have time, I recommend heading to Zuma, which is inside the Mandarin Oriental Hotel. It has an astonishing city view, and it's a great alternative for lovers of fusion cuisine…

ISTANBUL

FISH BY THE BOSPHORUS

I travel a lot for business, and everywhere I go, I try the cuisine. But what I miss the most about Istanbul, especially after long trips, is grilled fish by the Bosphorus... Nothing compares to some meze, followed by a good grilled fish, while gazing at the captivating view of the Bosphorus and Istanbul.

In reality, no meal is as easy as grilled fish! Buy some fresh fish, cook it and voilà! You don't need to work too hard. You don't need special sauces or side dishes. And there's no better gastronomical pleasure than eating fresh, grilled fish on a warm Istanbul evening by the sea. It's an experience that even outstrips the joy one experiences at a Michelin-starred restaurant. Of course, it's not all about the fish, because there's also the mezes in Istanbul. Italians and Spaniards have meze-like dishes, but you can't compare them with the whole meze experience in Turkey: Digging into meze and fish by the Bosphorus is something completely different.

I also have the habit of eating dessert after a good fish. I know this ritual sounds like calorific suicide, but a good balance of salad, meze and the best cornbread you'll ever taste in your life will make you feel better.

It's best to eat fish in Istanbul between April and October. If you eat in the fall and winter outside these times, you'll probably have to dine indoors – something that might knock the enjoyment factor down a peg or two. Above all, you don't get to see the perfect combination of the Bosphorus and perhaps the full moon in any other month. And if you don't believe me, just ask any foreign guest who's happened to experience such a night.

I have a couple of criteria regarding fish restaurants. For one, they need to be right by the sea – there can't be any intervening roads whatsoever. It's also important to have the option for indoor and outdoor dining. Above all, however, my overriding expectation is that the fish will be cooked appropriately: It can't be too dry or too raw; it has to be slightly moist in the middle.

Though you'll see that there are some places that do not meet some of these criteria, they're still on my list of favorites thanks to some other distinguishing qualities. As it is, I created this list – which, as always, is in alphabetical order – according to my own criteria and taste only, so I apologize to the regulars of any restaurant I haven't listed. I'm sure there are great restaurants that I haven't written about, especially as others might have escaped my attention, since I mostly go to the restaurants I know and love. If you have any of your own thoughts or recommendations, do let me know by email!

BALIKÇI ABDULLAH

Balıkçı Abdullah, located in Beykoz, is a beautiful restaurant that boasts well-cooked fish, mezes and good service. As I noted above, the most common mistake that Turkish fish restaurants make is to overdo the fish, leaving it dry. Abdullah, thankfully, understands what good fish is and knows how to cook it. Today, he rarely cooks (but he's always on hand to greet customers), but all the chefs in the restaurant were trained by him. The food and the service are also great; I, for one, keep coming back because of Abdullah's tarama (a Turkish/Greek meze), cornbread, fish and interesting meze.

In fact, cornbread and tarama tend to start off the evening, but be on your guard, because there's a risk of eating too much of them before you've even seen the meal to come. Now, the normal tradition is to choose your mezes from a tray that the waiter brings to your table, but at Balıkçı Abdullah, you may need to go to the kitchen to choose your mezes. Again, be careful, because you don't want to eat too much meze and miss out on some great fish! Nevertheless, make sure you have "lakerda" (bonito) – Abdullah just happens to serve the best in town.

There's a walking trail between the restaurant and the sea, which means that even if you grab the table closest to the water, there'll still be 3-5 meters between the sea and your table. Now, I prefer dining next to the sea in fish restaurants, but Balıkçı Abdullah has so many good qualities that I'll put these criteria aside. The restaurant has a big boat that departs from İstinye and brings you to the restaurant; just think, you can enjoy the Bosphorus for half an hour there and back, particularly when the weather is nice. Like I said, this is a joy you can't find anywhere else!

FERİYE
Feriye is a great place for meze. Diners can enjoy a view of the Ortaköy Mosque, as well as the Bosphorus Bridge, giving one a delightful, two-for-one panorama. They even have a glass greenhouse that allows you to dine by the sea, even during the winter.

Feriye is open every day from noon till midnight, so you can go there pretty much anytime, meaning that, if you're not in the mood for dinner, you could opt for Feriye's scrumptious breakfast on Saturdays and Sundays. The only downside is that Feriye tends to organize many weddings, meaning that if the wedding party is crowded, the kitchen tends to shift its focus there.

İSKELE

Located on a historical pier near Rumeli Hisari, İskele protrudes into the sea, offering you a vista of the Bosphorus on three sides. İskele (whose very name means pier) has good fish and meze. Regrettably, they don't have an outdoor dining area; come summer, they do open the windows, but that's just not the same as dining al fresco. Still, the view of Anadolu Hisari across the water on the Asian side is beautiful.

Moreover, the boats going to some of the top fish restaurants on the Asian side, Lacivert and Uskumru, also depart from the vicinity, meaning that if you're ever in the neighborhood, you have three different fish restaurant options!

A DIFFERENT FISH FOR EVERY SEASON

In many restaurants abroad, you can order fish on the menu almost all year round. Every fish, however, has a season. For example, bonito is good in September, bluefish is best in October, large bluefish goes in November and turbot is in season come December and January... Why would one eat sea bass all year when you can eat different – and better – fish every season?

KIYI

Kıyı is a restaurant like no other for me; after all, I've been going there for the past 45 years. There used to be a lot of traveling photographers in these kinds of places. They'd take a photo of a person and give it to them afterwards in a little folder. Now, when I look through my old photo albums, I see how many pictures there are of me at Kıyı. I even had my college graduation dinner there! Thirty years ago, Kıyı, like many other fish restaurants, used to put tables on the other side of the road by the sea, allowing you to dine with the water lapping up against the shore around your shoes. Unfortunately, they don't do this anymore, but it's still one of Istanbul's oldest survivors, and it's one of the oldest restaurant on my list. And 50 years on, Kıyı's owner is still running the place, just like he was half a century ago. Through the years, the taste has remained the same, that is, excellent. Their pickles are to die for, as are the beans, liver, calamari, home-made salted bonito and very fresh fish.

LACİVERT

Lacivert is located on the Asian side of Istanbul, right beneath the second Bosphorus Bridge and directly across from İskele. Both Lacivert and its next-door neighbor, Uskumru, have boats, so you can use marine transportation to arrive at one of these restaurants if you'd like.

Lacivert's cook has been working here for years; he travels abroad and goes to seminars, meaning he can cook many interesting dishes besides traditional Turkish cuisine. A place with a large, international clientele, Lacivert is a chic restaurant with a cozy environment in which you can peacefully eat meze and fish. You can sip a drink at the bar and even listen to live jazz music sometimes.

And like Feriye, it's a good spot for breakfast on the weekends.

The view, on the other hand, is unreal, with spectacular vistas of the First Bridge. Lacivert has a long strip of coastline on the shore, giving it a number of tables right next to the sea. Lacivert also has a wine cellar that features about 200 types of wine, about half of which are probably foreign (by contrast, none of the other places on today's list have such a cellar). If you have a visitor who's interested in wine, then this is the place to go.

MARİNA BALIK

I've been going to Marina, located inside Kuruçeşme Park on Istanbul's European side, for a couple of years. They have an area outdoors, but I don't recommend it, as the indoor area is the one that's actually on the sea. Come summer, they open the glass windows, allowing you to soak in the sea. It's an elegant restaurant thanks to its service, tablecloths and napkins.

USKUMRU

An elegant restaurant next to Lacivert, Uskumru is a place that mostly cooks traditional Turkish meals. What Uskumru lacks in a long shore like Lacivert it more than makes up for with its talented chef, who happens to make two delicious types of cornbread, pan-cooked and oven-baked. Uskumru's salted bonito is also extra tasty, as are their original salads, grilled octopus and calamari.

Mind you, I only visit Uskumru (and Lacivert, for that matter) if I can eat outside, as their respective interior sections are too far away from the sea. (In contrast, the interior sections at Feriye, İskele and Marina are all close by the water.) And lest you forget, Uskumru and Lacivert both provide marine transportation, meaning you can get to the European side with a hop, skip and a jump.

YENİKÖY ALEKO

The owner of Aleko in Yeniköy might have changed, but the new owner has preserved the name and the cuisine of the place. Aleko is a modernized version of an old Greek taverna where they open the glass windows during the summer to let in the sea breeze. Most of the waiters are around 40 or 50, and have been there since the place opened many years ago. They prepare delicious fish and meze, and the service is great.

TRİLYE

Trilye isn't open yet, but I hope it will be soon. When it does, it's bound to be one of the best fish restaurants in Istanbul. I went to a high school in Bebek, and we would sometimes go to a restaurant called Güneş when we could afford to go. The place – 50 years ago now – had a view of the Bay of Bebek and sported old wooden chairs and tables. In time, the owner changed, renaming it Yeni Güneş. The prices rose, as did the quality of the tables and chairs, but I kept going there. Later, they also expanded the terrace and moved it slightly toward the sea. Fifteen years ago, the owner changed again, renaming it Poseidon and launching operations with some of the old waiters. The tables changed, tablecloths appeared, new dishes found their way onto the menu and a better wine cellar soon developed. It closed a couple of years ago, but now they say that new owners from Ankara are soon to open up the place again after making a deal with the famous Trilye. Given that the location has such a special place in my heart, I can't wait.

ANKARA

Trilye is a wonderful restaurant in Ankara that cooks fish to an Istanbul quality. Even if I'm in Ankara just for the day, I always visit Trilye, where there's always fresh fish and meze on the menu. On top of that, the owner really strives to make a difference here. He's always at work, both cooking and serving. Trilye will soon open doors at the old Poseidon in Istanbul, bringing together the memories of Güneş, Yeni Güneş, Poseidon and Trilye.

But when one says Ankara, one of the other fish restaurants that immediately comes to mind is Kalbur. If I'm staying in Ankara for a night, then I'll probably have a meal at Trilye and another at little Kalbur. These two restaurants have completely different styles, yet they both cook great fish. It's just a couple that runs Kalbur: one cooks, the other serves. I've asked the owners why they don't open an Istanbul branch, but they just answer that they can hardly deal with the restaurant in Ankara! Given that, I reckon we'll have to content ourselves with a journey to the capital if we're to enjoy the tastes of Kalbur.

FISH ON AN ISLAND

Besides eating fish by the Bosphorus, you can also dig into some seafood on one of the Prince Islands. All five islands are home to hundreds of fish restaurants along their long shorelines. The islands are very busy on the weekends, when eateries tend to focus their efforts.

For this reason, the places have become pretty touristy, meaning waiters will often be pretty insistent that you sit down to eat if you happen to be walking past the front. Most of the island restaurants bring fish from markets in Istanbul rather than procuring them from fishermen on the island. Still, there's a really nice, small, family restaurant on Burgaz Island that I like, Fincan, which is run by Canan and Rasim. Canan is incredibly talented in the kitchen, while her husband, Rasim, is skilled in service.

You can eat all day in Fincan, from breakfast to dinner. Canan prepares around 40 types of meze depending on the season, but they serve up tasty international meze as well. Moreover, they cook the fish really well – although I usually forego the fish at Fincan just so I can sample all the meze. Note, though, that their wine list is limited.

Even if you go to another of the islands, I would recommend you stop by on Burgaz for some dinner at Fincan. There's also an ice cream place nearby which, I think, has the best ice cream in all of Istanbul. Go get an ice cream after a dinner at Fincan and, as they say in Turkish, "kill the fish."

THREE CHEF-OWNED ISTANBUL RESTAURANTS WITH GREAT FISH

It's never entirely clear why, but new restaurants in Istanbul often close very quickly. Even very good brands end up having to close down places. Ultimately, a restaurant stays open only if international customers become regulars – that's because Turkish customers have the habit of getting bored with a restaurant they like. International customers, on the other hand, are more loyal.

At the same time, there's a new trend in which the owner of a restaurant doubles as the chef which, in my view, is a great thing.

MIKLA

At Mehmet Gürs' Mikla, everything is local and nothing is frozen. One of Turkey's top restaurants, Mikla offers a three-course meal and a six-course one, one of which can be vegetarian.

Mikla's cooks, too, are always on their feet, as just seven cook for the 140 guests that dine from 6 p.m. to midnight.

The wine list is approved by Wine Spectator and features top Turkish varieties. Add in the best view in town, as well as perfect service, and you absolutely can't go wrong with Mikla.

NEOLOKAL

The old headquarters of Istanbul's Ottoman Bank, which is now owned by Garanti Bank, is known for its unique architecture. The place is currently home to a library and museum called Salt Galata, as well as a restaurant called Neolokal, run by chef/owner Maksut

Askar. When Neolokal took over the restaurant from the previous owners, an Italian restaurant called Ca d'Oro, they changed everything but the kitchen and the decorations, transforming the place. The owner, the chef, his team and the menu all changed completely.

The restaurant serves Turkish meals – with a unique take – and is open every day except Monday. You can order meze and down some rakı if you like. I think Neolokal will be a successful restaurant – the only downside is that it's a bit remote for Turkish customers. On another note, there is a simple café in the same building that's perfect for the peckish library and museum visitor.

WORLD-RENOWNED CAN ROCA COOKED IN THIS RESTAURANT

Sponsored by Garanti Bank, the famous Spanish restaurant Can Roca – the world's best restaurant in 2015 – came to Turkey for a brilliant food event. Can Rosa used Neolokal's kitchen to cook and also made use of Neolokal's chefs, providing an excellent opportunity for some knowledge transfer. I've learned that one or two Neolokal chefs will go to Can Roca for some training; it's a great opportunity for Turkish chefs!

YENİ LOKANTA

Civan Er, who used to work in Muzedechanga, opened his own restaurant in Beyoğlu, dubbing it Yeni Lokanta (New Restaurant). Er cooks fusion Turkish food, with some of the dishes greatly resembling the ones he used to cook at Muzedechanga, while others are completely new. Nevertheless, you'll taste the elements of Turkish cuisine in whatever you eat. Er is a chef who's always at work; he mostly spends his time in the kitchen, but you can also see him with customers as well.

Transportation by car is difficult, but the walking distance is not too far for those who are fond of walking on the vibrant streets of Beyoğlu. A place with a simple design, Yeni Lokanta doesn't have a wide range of wines on their menu, although you can find many Turkish wines. Yeni Lokanta is a great place to try different interpretations of traditional Turkish food, including mezes and fresh fish. It's also the perfect place to entertain foreign guests thanks to Beyoğlu's impressive atmosphere.

KOYOTO

East Asia is a different world in every way. Ever astonishing, the region perpetually has a surprise in store for the visitor. But among the region's many features, I'm mostly interested in their spectacular cuisine…

THREE MICHELIN STARS FOR A SEVEN-SEAT RESTAURANT

Osaka and Kyoto are connected by a high-speed train that zips along at a brisk 240 km/h, meaning that a journey that once took an hour now takes a mere 15 minutes.

We stayed in the city for two days, dining in two different restaurants during our sojourn. Our first reservation was for a restaurant called Chihana. It's a tiny place that sits just seven people – three at the sushi bar and four more at the tables. A gentleman and a lady own the place: The lady serves, while the gentleman prepares the sushi. For drinks, there are champagne, or red or white wine; you can choose one of them. (We opted for the champagne, deeming it the least risky option.)

At Chihana, all the dishes are prepared in front of you. The chef, who is clearly a professional, cut and cleaned a shrimp that was more than jumbo size right before our eyes. The chef also prepared more than 20 kinds of sushi, sashimi and rolls. He has a style all his own – a style that is impressive enough for Japanese standards that it fetched three Michelin stars. In a nutshell, the meal was delicious but very costly!

THREE MICHELIN STARS FOR A SIX-TABLE RESTAURANT

The night after Chihana, we went to Kitcho Arashiyama, a famous restaurant where customers have to make a reservation six months in advance. Because I had previously tried but failed to make a reservation for the place, it wasn't even on our Kyoto itinerary. But as luck would have it, Kitcho Arashiyama informed us while we were in Kyoto that we could make a reservation for lunch – an opportunity we were certainly not going to turn down. The restaurant is a full 50-minute drive from the city, but that didn't stop us; along the way, we even got a chance to see some up the rest of the prefecture.

Like Chihana, Kitcho Arashiyama is run by a husband-wife team in which the man cooks and the woman serves. Kitcho Arashiyama is also an intriguing establishment with six rooms, each of which has just a single table. In other words, the whole place has just six tables, none of which see each other. In keeping with Japanese culture, we sat on the floor, deciding what to eat with the help of the server. The food was out of this world, while the whole evening had an aura of yesteryear. At the end of our meal, the owner of the restaurant served us dessert.

A PIECE OF ADVICE

There's no hotel that I would particularly recommend staying at in Kyoto, as I didn't think ours was particularly up to scratch. That said, hotels in the area – including ours – can offer the services of a good, English-speaking driver to see the sights in both Osaka and Kyoto. This is indeed what we did in Kyoto, and it turned out to be a nice experience, as our driver proved to be informative throughout the ride. The drivers can ferry you to local museums and, more importantly, find ways to evade the lineup to get in.

LONDON

One of the cities that I and my friends from the Turkish business world visit the most is London. For me, though, it's not all about work, as I also travel there often just for vacation.

But without further ado, here are my top 10 London restaurants, listed in alphabetical order.

1. COYA

Coya is a new Peruvian restaurant that mainly serves seafood – a staple of the country's cuisine – and vegetarian fare. Being on the ground floor, it doesn't have much in the way of a view, so it's best to head there for dinner. At least, though, you can enjoy the lively, Peruvian décor on the walls. The restaurant sets out common dishes and then you just help yourself. The restaurant, with a seating capacity of 200, has a bar upstairs that offers live music, so you may as well go there for a few drinks or a coffee afterward.

2. DINNER BY HESTON

Dinner By Heston is the name of the restaurant that Heston Blumenthal started inside the Mandarin Oriental Hotel in London. I once had a lunch appointment with an important customer of mine and wanted to take him to the restaurant. But try as I might (twice, in fact), I couldn't land a booking for my preferred date. In my hour of need, I turned to İsa Bal, the sommelier of the Fat Duck, Heston Blumenthal's first restaurant, for help. İsa was able to open doors, and I finally went there with my guest.

The system at Dinner by Heston is different

than that of the Fat Duck, as Blumenthal continues to serve a 17-course menu at his first location. For Dinner By Heston, it appears that he has employed his own right-hand person, Ashley Palmer, as executive chef. About 10-12 chefs cook in a tiny glass room that resembles an aquarium; it might make the cooks feel like they're in a fishbowl, but it allows you to watch your food being prepared.

Another great thing is that all of the dishes here are drawn from the cuisine of Medieval England. The menu includes the history of the dish, as well as further elaborate information about how it was cooked. Dinner By Heston has a simpler menu compared to the Fat Duck, but the beauty of this place is that it is open every single day, including Sundays. What's more, it has a great view of Hyde Park!

3. FAT DUCK

Now in his 50s, Heston Blumenthal is the chef, founder, owner and, in short, jack of all trades of the Fat Duck, which is located in Bray, about a 45-minute drive from London. You should go for the tasting menu at the Fat Duck which is itself situated within a historical building that can sit around 80 people. The tasting menu is a four-hour affair, so I reckon it's best to go there at noon, if possible, as the menu might prove to be too heavy for dinner. And if you go there during the day, you'll have the opportunity to tour about the pretty town and its centuries-old buildings.

Another thing to note is that the Fat Duck has a Turkish sommelier, İsa Bal, a well-trained specialist in winemaking. On top of that, he's acquired his Master of Wine qualification, which is doled out by a council of world-famous enologists that test applicants once or twice a year. If candidates pass a written exam, they are then subjected to an oral one, as well as a tasting test. Successful candidates are then accepted to the council as fellow brothers. Altogether, it takes years to acquire the distinction of Master of Wine.

The wine menu in Fat Duck is as thick as a phone book; it really is all-inclusive. Beyond that, a Blumenthal plate also appeals to all five senses: In addition to tasting it, you hear it crunch in your mouth, smell it, see it and touch it.

Blumenthal has also written several cookbooks that feature recipes on various types of food. Here though, they use "Sous Vide," the technique of low-temperature cooking, so as not to lose any nutrients. All the food is cooked at around 70 to 85 degrees so that it won't boil. After that, they place the food in vacuumed bags, which are then put into hot water at a preheated temperature.

4. GORDON RAMSAY

One of the most famous British chefs in the world, Gordon Ramsay is a man who owns restaurants around the globe, even though he doesn't cook anymore. Ramsay, of course, is a notoriously angry chef that treats his staff horrendously. And before he was a cook, he even claims to have played in the first team of Rangers in the Scottish Premier League.

In London, he was once the cook of the illustrious restaurant Aubergine. I tried to make a reservation there once, but they were only accepting bookings for six months in advance – and charging up front to boot. Nevertheless, I did make a reservation this way, only for the man himself to leave Aubergine to open a new restaurant in Chelsea named after himself. I duly canceled my previous reservation at Aubergine to book a table at Gordon Ramsay's new Gordon Ramsay.

The restaurant known as Gordon Ramsay is a cramped establishment next to the street that can sit 45 people. It's a good place for both lunch and dinner, although like all places in London, its lunch menu is somewhat cheaper. Boasting three Michelin stars, the restaurant displays a particular understanding of food presentation and design. And as a popular and award-winning public figure, Gordon Ramsey also sells his cookbooks in the restaurant.

But here's another word to the wise: When truffles are in season, the restaurant offers a wide selection of truffles. Also, anyone that wants to get their hands a bit dirty can take a cooking lesson with an advance reservation and help the cooks prep from 9:30 a.m. to 12:30 p.m.

5. LA PETITE MAISON

With branches in Nice, London, Dubai, Istanbul and Beirut, La Petit Maison is a fine French Mediterranean restaurant that serves up a characteristic cuisine. Along with its French fare, it shares some similarities with Zuma and Roka in that it serves dishes in the Japanese izakaya style of dining; that is, the dishes are brought one after another to the table and shared. In that, it actually suits our dining customs as well.

Although it's a French restaurant, the executive chef is Raphael, who hails from Nigeria. Interestingly, he doesn't seem to use any butter in his cooking;

instead, he leans heavily on olive oil, salad and fish. The restaurant certainly has the influences of Italy and Southern France, but it might be more appropriate to call the food Mediterranean. The dishes served here include socca with Côte d'Azur origins, pissaladière, Italian burrata, mozzarella, marinated raw fish, green lentils and bulgur salad.

6. MARCUS WAREING
Following a bitter falling-out with Gordon Ramsay, Marcus Wareing left his job as head chef of the aforementioned restaurant Gordon Ramsay to open his own establishment, which, appropriately enough, is called Marcus Wareing. (Wareing said he will never speak to Ramsay against in his life, but admitted that he does admire the celebrity chef's cooking.)

Wareing's two-star restaurant, which is located in the Berkeley Hotel, is extremely comfortable and roomy. It also offers somewhat affordable pricing for lunch.

The restaurant's chefs tend to use a considerable amount of vegetables and herbs in their cooking. And one more thing: There is also a chef's table for eight that gives you a perfect glimpse into the kitchen while you're eating.

7. NOBU
Nobu, owned in part by Robert De Niro, has 30 locations worldwide, 10 of which I've managed to eat at. Of these, my favorite is the Nobu right below the Metropolitan Hotel in London, thanks to its wonderful view over Hyde Park and the variety on its menu.

The owner was born in Japan, but he lived for

many years in Peru – something that gives the cuisine a notable Peruvian influence. The place even has sushi of his own invention, a factor that makes him a god among Japanese sushi chefs.

8. OBLIX

Oblix was founded in London on the 32nd floor of the Shard, the highest building in Europe. Oblix's cuisine ranges from French to German to American. And as you would expect given its location, it has a splendid 360-degree view of London, as well as live jazz music.

9. ROKA

Situated on Charlotte Street in central London, Roka is a two-storied restaurant. It's got a Robata grill setup on the first floor, where nearly 120 people can dine. They also have an al fresco dining area for 40 on sunny days. On the ground floor is a bar that is livelier in the evenings. The section, where you can both eat and drink, gives one the general impression that you're at a nightclub. The bar, which also offers live music, is ideal for parties of 40-50 people.

Heading the Roka empire is a Kiwi cook, Amish. Right now, Roka has two locations in London, as well as another in Hong Kong, but there are plans to open two more restaurants in London in the near future. Although Roka resembles Zuma, it's more contemporary and less expensive.

10. ZUMA

Zuma now has many branches worldwide, but the very first – and still one of the very best – is located in

London. (The locations in Miami and Dubai give the London branch a run for its money, while there are also branches in Hong Kong, Abu Dhabi, New York and Istanbul.)

Zuma was co-founded by an Indian entrepreneur, Arjun Waney, and an experienced German chef, Rainer Becker, who learned to specialize in Japanese cuisine when he worked in Tokyo some years ago. The location can currently serve up to 250 customers at a time using Robata-style grilling. Open seven days a week, Zuma serves both lunch and dinner, yet it's always a good idea to make a reservation, because it's a popular place.

As for the seating style, you can eat around a table, at the sushi bar or even at the grill. It offers a wide range of dazzling dishes from sushi to grilled food, while the wine menu is brilliant too. And the sommelier, Alessandro, is simply the real deal.

When Londoners were asked their reasons for going to restaurants, they listed the ambiance, the ability to socialize, the chance to enjoy themselves and only then, in fourth place, did they list the food. That is to say, one doesn't simply go to a restaurant to eat one's fill: Zuma, thankfully, fits the bill for everything on the list.

MACAU

East Asia is a different world in every which way. The region always astonishes me – as well as everyone else. It'll be no surprise to you, though, that one of the things that interests me most about East Asia is its spectacular cuisine…

If you're planning a trip to the Far East, you might as well spend a few days in Macau – the Las Vegas of the region, so to speak. (In fact, Macau even has more machines and casinos than Sin City.) The city's gambling culture is the main reason behind the existence of its large and luxurious hotels, one of which is the Grand Hyatt Hotel, a new and eminently chic building. The Grand Hyatt doesn't lack for machines to gamble, while it also has a nice performance center. Make sure you don't miss the interesting shows performed every evening.

The Eight, a Chinese restaurant located in the Grand Lisboa Hotel, is extremely inviting with its three Michelin stars. The place probably has the largest wine menu I have ever seen; no lie, they probably have 100,000 bottles of at least 1,500 different wines.

With so many wines to choose from, they've developed an innovative system for ordering: a tablet application. When you want to choose your wine, a waiter brings you a tablet. You enter your preferences and, presto, the app spits out appropriate suggestions. For example, if you'd like a 2000 vintage Bordeaux for under 300 dollars, the app will show you all the wines available at the restaurant that match your criteria. It's a great way to go about ordering some wine!

MELBOURNE

Melbourne offers a different type of beauty to its eternal Australian rival, Sydney. It's a happy place with a large student population, beaches and lots of places to wine and dine. Even if Melbourne isn't as touristy as Sydney, it's a city that needs to be visited in its own right. A metropolis of 4.5 million people, Melbourne is an hour-long flight away from Sydney. From what Australians say, Melbourne is the continent's most enjoyable and easygoing city.

And if you ask the foreigners that also live here, they'd say the same thing. Many university students choose Melbourne as their place of study, including many Americans, thanks to educational institutions that are some of the best in the world. And even if the Americans have perhaps the best 15 universities in the world, the price of an Australian university is just a quarter of its U.S. counterpart. In fact, I met an American student here who was helping to pay for tuition by driving for Uber – he seemed to really like living here.

While Sydney resembles more New York Midtown or the area around Central Park, Melbourne is more akin to Soho Tribeca – and it seems a bit more like Europe. In terms of urban planning, Melbourne also appears to have had more success.

But I digress, we're here for Melbourne's restaurants! Here they are, again in alphabetical order.

ATTICA
It's well-nigh impossible to find a seat at this Australian restaurant, which is among the cream of the

crop near the top of the world's top 50 list. In the end, we had Mehmet Gürs' intervention to thank for allowing us to make a reservation, although it wasn't under the most ideal of circumstances: We had to be there at 6 p.m. – not my most preferred time – and out by 8:30 p.m. Attica has a set menu for all; the only possible alteration is to choose fish if you don't eat meat. Nonetheless, we reckoned that it would be impossible to come all the way to Melbourne and not go to Attica. The prices truly are astronomical, but boy was the food out of this world. It was the best meal I had in Melbourne, but more than that, if I were on the jury to vote for the world's best restaurant, I think I'd probably vote for Attica. We had a 12-course menu, 10 of which we enjoyed. I had no complaints because I opted to go meat-free, although my daughter did not. Ultimately, that meant that she had to dine out on fried ant (probably for the first and last time), which is consumed in Australia. If you're not interested in ingesting delicacies like this, it's a good idea to sometimes put a limit on the meat. In any case, even if Attica has been selected as Australia's best restaurant, it's good to be on your guard. In the end, though, I think I would still opt for Sydney's Bennelong over Attica – although my decision might be impacted by the fact that I'm not a big fan of the inflexibility of set menus.

CUMULUS UP

Cumulus Up is a two-floor affair. In actuality, the bottom floor is known just as Cumulus, while the upper floor – hence the "up" – is the actual eatery in question. The bottom floor, which doesn't take reservations (if you can find a seat, you get to sit), has a pub atmosphere that's geared toward fun. The top floor, however, requires reservations. When you do order, you can do everything at once or item by item. We headed to Cumulus Up for an enjoyable reunion with Sera, the daughter of Barış Tansever, the owner of the well-regarded Istanbul restaurant Sunset. Thanks to Sera's knowledge of the Melbourne food scene (she's currently studying in the city), we ordered ourselves some excellent food. While the two women plumped for meat, I, as always, opted for seafood. In the accompaniment of an American wine, we had ourselves a wonderful Australian fusion feast.

EMBLA

Embla is a popular, lunch-oriented wine bar that's in the heart of the city. Customers can order from an hors d'oeuvres menu that features tapas-like offerings of Australian food. Embla serves great Australian wine, and – this is the best bit – they do it in the right glasses at the right temperature. Because it's located in the city center, Embla is easy to reach (a factor which no doubt increases the number of customers). In the end, Embla is a perfect place to escape for some wine and food for Melbourne's white-collar workers, who make up the vast majority of the clientele. It also has reasonable prices that are in line with what you would get in Cihangir. Note, though, that you're unlikely to find the same jovial atmosphere in the evenings.

ROOFTOP AT QT
Located in one of Melbourne's few tall buildings,

Rooftop at QT really is a place you need to visit at night. Take a seat and enjoy the view of Melbourne stretching toward the sea alongside some light food and wine or beer (the country, naturally, also has excellent beer). When you go to the bar to order your drinks, you can also order your tapas-like hors d'oeuvres. After paying, they'll give you a number for your table and bring it your food when it's ready. And if you're interested in some more food, you do the same routine again. All this means that waiters aren't taking your orders – perhaps because it's cheaper for the establishment. A place that leaves everyone with a pleasant feeling, Rooftop at QT is a bar for people who are just getting off work, as well as for ever-chatty Melburnians looking to socialize.

TOP MEDOC

Top Medoc is a breakfast eatery opened by a horse-racing fanatic. I say breakfast place, but Top Medoc does serve lunch and dinner. Founded on healthy food, turmeric, egg whites, chia, wheatgrass juice, ginger and other such ingredients are all front and center at Top Medoc. For drinks, they serve things like coffee with almond milk and coconut juice. Really, everything you've ever heard about healthy eating is to be found here, so don't bother trying to order meat, sausage or bacon (although you might be able to get a piece of smoked salmon on top of egg). If you happened to have overdone it on food the day before, Top Medoc is the perfect place for a detox the day after.

YARRA VALLEY DAIRY

The last place I want to recommend in Melbourne is actually outside the city; more than that, it's actually a farm – albeit one with a restaurant attached. If you want to get into the car, get out of town and spend some time in nature, look no further than Yarra Valley Dairy. The valley itself has two large wine houses where they both grow their own grapes and make their own wine. Of course, you can visit these as well, but I want to talk about the farm. The Yarra Valley Farm raises sheep, goats and cows to make cheese, which the on-site restaurant serves alongside local wine. Actually, though, that's not really doing it justice, because their menu also boasts fresh, crunchy bread and olive oil produced on the farm. Like at Rooftop at QT, you make your selection, pay for your food and take a number to your table. After they bring your food, the only thing that you have to do is eat and take in the wonderful nature. In summer, they might offer service outside as well, which, you can sure, would also be an experience to savor.

If you're interested in going to the farm, you ought to set aside five or six hours. And as far as I'm concerned, the best idea is to agree with a driver so that you can squeeze out all the enjoyment you can from the journey. I would suggest first touring the valley, then visiting one of the art galleries at the wine houses and, finally, topping it off with a feast of fantastic of cheese and wine at the Yarra Valley Dairy. And there's also a zoo where you can see some of the area's snakes, alligators and kangaroos. Don't miss it!

BEWARE!

According to old English lore, you should only have fish in months that contain an "R," meaning it's fine to have them from September to April. The folk wisdom, however, is only valid for the Northern Hemisphere (and even then, it's more for those who like raw fish), as the "R" months are spread over summer in the south, meaning that it might be good to steer clear of tuna sashimi when it's so hot out and bacteria can grow more quickly. And even if you cook the fish, the center might remain uncooked. Above all, eating bad shellfish like mussels and oysters can make you sick for four or five days. Just something to think about when you lose yourself in the Fish Market...

MILAN

Trussardi is a fashion brand popular the world over among men and women.

Trussardi, however, isn't just in the clothing business; it also has a restaurant on the top floor of its shop in Milan. Ristorante Trussardi Alla Scala has seating for around 70 to 80 people, boasts a couple of Michelin stars and serves up a delectable mix of fusion cuisine. You might not be able to find the most standard Italian dishes, but the taste of the food is not too far off from Italian cuisine. It has a rich menu that includes several types of risotto, macaroni and ossobuco. Everything is Italian, albeit with a little bit of reinterpretation.

People who come here to shop generally stop to have lunch at the restaurant or in the café. Come evening, the place mostly becomes the haunt of businesspeople. But as the restaurant's full name might suggest, its most important feature is its proximity to La Scala.

If you're keen on going, you must book a reservation a couple of days ahead of time.

But while I'm at it, let me suggest a hotel for your stay in Milan. The Park Hyatt is just a short hop, skip and a jump from Trussardi. Located inside a historical building, the Park Hyatt has high ceilings – something that I really like. The bathrooms, too, are as wide as the rooms.

The Park Hyatt has been around for about 10 years now. They also have a nice restaurant that's suitable for both lunch and dinner.

MODENA

One of the world's 10 best restaurants, there's no place quite like Osteria Francescana in Modena. Well-worth its three Michelin stars, it offers fairly modern Italian cuisine.

The restaurant's capacity, however, is as small as its reputation is big. The osteria has one dining room for 10 people, as well as another one for 20 people – ultimately meaning it's difficult to find a place at one of the individual tables.

If you do snag a place, may I suggest you try the gastronomical menu. But if you're pressed for time, try for three or four dishes. The dishes are served as small, non-fusion portions.

Francescana goes for the minimal in its decoration, although it does have pink walls.

The restaurant is also located in an alley, which can cause problems, especially as the area is closed to traffic on the weekends, meaning you might need to stretch your legs a bit if you're arriving by car on Saturday or Sunday.

But while Osteria Francescana has gained fame in the world, Modena's hotels are not similarly up to scratch, as I couldn't find any worth staying in.

NEW YORK

I travel to New York for a whole host of reasons. But whatever my reason for going to the Big Apple, whenever I go, I try and visit as many restaurants as possible, including whatever is new on the scene.

I've written about New York's restaurants before, but much water has since passed under the bridge; in the intervening time, some restaurants have been closed, while others have lowered their standards. More than that, though, writing again provides me the chance to run the rule over a whole bunch of new restaurants.

As always, I've listed all the restaurants in alphabetical order. All the places below are personal choices, but if you have your own restaurant experiences or recommendations you'd like to share, please email me at metinar@metinar.com.

BLUE HILL AT STONE BARNS

Not many people know this restaurant, which is about 50 minutes out of town by cab in Stone Barns at a ranch that was, interestingly, built by Rockefeller. Here, they grow all kinds of organic vegetables and raise pigs, chicken and small cows. I don't generally deign to eat eggs, but I definitely did here.

Everything looks good, smells nice and tastes even better, probably because of the fodder they use. All the meals, apart from the fish, are prepared with the freshest of ingredients that are produced right on the farm. Blue Hill's chef, Dan Barber, has been in charge of the kitchen since day one. You can enjoy a dinner at Blue Hill six days a week, while there is also an additional lunch service on Saturdays and Sundays. This being the United States, dinner begins as early as 5:30 p.m., so I recommend you make a reservation for as early in the evening as possible. More than that, try and go an hour early, because it's a lot of fun to spend time both in the town and the farm. (And don't be tardy about planning your trip to Blue Hill either: Reservations are a big problem at the restaurant, but if you send an email at least five or six weeks in advance and are flexible about time, you'll get results.)

A spacious and calm place with 10-meter-high ceilings, Blue Hill can host 50 people. Thankfully, the tables are spread out from one another, allowing you to chat comfortably. Blue Hill also has a splendid wine menu, which has offerings from all over the world at a good price. At your typical fine restaurant, the wines are priced at a wholesale price multiplied by around four; at Blue Hill, however, they only multiply this price by two, even though it's a top restaurant. More than that, you can order wines by the glass, giving you the opportunity to taste a different wine for every dish if you plan to try five or six different things. On top of that, all the waiters at Blue Hill are very knowledgeable about food and wine. And while most New York restaurants typically have a high circulation in terms of waiters, almost of Blue Hill's wait staff has been there since the first day.

The restaurant's chef, Dan Barber, used to be former U.S. President Barack Obama's nutrition consultant. Barber also made it onto Time's "Time 100" list in 2009. The influential chef's farmers decide what's on the menu that day: "I shape a menu based on the products that the farmers bring. I can also prepare personalized menus for guests," says Barber. There's another Blue Hill in Manhattan with similar menus, but I recommend the one in Stone Barns.

ELEVEN MADISON PARK

Eleven Madison Park was named the world's best restaurant in 2017. I wasn't impressed the first time I went there for lunch, but boy was I charmed by their dinner service the second time I went. From 7:30 p.m. to 11:30 p.m., our group of four had a wonderful meal. First of all, there is no menu here; instead, our waiter chatted with us to find out about what we like and don't like. Armed with this information, they prepared personal menus consisting of 15 dishes. I had fish, while my friends had meat and veggies. And all through the meal, chefs and waiters swung by our table to tell us the stories of each of our dishes. Moreover, there was a trick, a touch in every plate. It was just like a cabaret... It was most certainly an exciting and enjoyable dinner.

The place, which can host 50-60 people, boasts church-like high ceilings that create a sense of comfort. The tables are also distant from one another, which spares you some of the noise from the other tables. And in my humble opinion, the wine menu is also great. It's usually a tall order trying to find half-bottles of wine on the menu, but Eleven Madison Park is one of those rare places (it's also something that allows them to serve a number of good brands). We, for one, had a half-bottle of the famous and rare Petrus for, appropriately enough, half the price of a normal Petrus, although we also tried different wines with every dish.

Eleven Madison Park is ultimately a place where you can let go and just enjoy yourself.

JUNGSIK

ungsik is a Korean restaurant that my friend brought me to one day. I loved it so much that I went to visit it again the next time I was in the Big Apple. This time, though, I had to make a reservation; in the intervening two years, they had picked up two Michelin stars, giving them a tremendous boost in popularity.

I don't have vast knowledge of Korean cuisine, but Jungsik's fare was quite different from what I've had before in South Korea. It's clear that they've made a fusion – and a perfect one at that – of Korean and Western cuisine, to the degree that if the waiters weren't Korean, you might not know that this is a Korean restaurant at all. Adapting a cuisine to another is a challenging thing to do; that's why we mostly see reinterpretations, such as Mehmet Gürs' Mikla, a Turkish restaurant reinterpreting traditional Turkish food in Istanbul.

A great alternative for fine dining, Jungsik is a modern restaurant with a top-notch wine menu. Besides the à la carte menu, they have two tasting menus, one of which is larger than the others. I recommend you try at least one of these tasting menus. If you have ingredients or dishes that you'd rather not have with the tasting menu, they change it as per your request.

LE BERNARDIN

One of the first places that comes to mind when you say food and New York is Le Bernardin. Gilbert and

Mathilde Le Coze opened the famous fish restaurant first in Paris in 1972 before raising the curtain on a second branch in New York 14 years later. Gilbert, who was also the chef, passed away shortly after the opening, giving way to Eric Ripert, one of his associates. Although the cuisine is French in origin, it is quite Americanized today.

In my opinion, Le Bernardin is the best fish restaurant in New York – everyone should eat there at least once! If you go there for lunch, you can have a beautiful fish menu in a very comfortable environment for a lower price than usual. Normally, I don't like the service of three-Michelin-star restaurants because of their attitude, but Le Bernardin is one such restaurant with three Michelin stars that has great service. Try to make reservations one week in advance.

LOCANDA VERDE

An Italian-American restaurant, Locanda Verde is located inside a hotel in Soho, although it has its own entrance as well. Open from noon to night, Verde can become a bit crowded around 8 p.m., when it gets busy for dinner service, but reservations aren't much of a problem otherwise. They have a very simple and modern menu consisting of at least 40 dishes. They also offer good service.

MAREA

A popular haunt for businessmen, Marea is another Italian restaurant overlooking Central Park's southwest corner on Columbus Circle, where New York's best restaurants are located. I can confidently say that Marea is the best Italian restaurant outside Italy, with everything done to Italian standards. If you visit Marea in October or November, you can find seven or eight dishes — including eggs – prepared with white truffles. When you're at Marea, you truly feel like you're dining at a high-quality restaurant in Rome. The place has two Michelin stars, but it's a question of when, not if, it gets a third. Marea is an expensive restaurant, but it's worth shelling out for a meal. They also have a nice bar that's great for a few drinks before dinner. And as with many other New York restaurants, you can eat for a lower price at lunch – meaning it might be a good idea to go there at midday, even if the menu is a bit more limited. Still, don't forget to make a reservation, just in case.

A DAYTIME VIEW OF CENTRAL PARK
If you're just visiting New York for a couple of days, you'll surely want to experience its food scene. If you have a few more days – and you're hankering after a proper taste of Italy – then look no further than Marea. If you want to survey all the beauty that is Central Park, it's best to head to Marea for lunch.

MORTON'S STEAKHOUSE
Morton's Steakhouse is a classic American chain. As you know, there are many steakhouses in New York, but there's none like Morton's for me. And here's one little tidbit to keep in mind at Morton's: The moment you sit, they serve the whitest and hottest bread in the world – right out of the oven! As if that isn't enough, they also bring olive oil and butter in large cups. Getting hungrier every minute, you end up ordering way too many. The moral of the story? Don't devour

too many and run out of room for what you actually came here for. Just remember to think about all the things you can order and distance yourself from the bread.

They have around 10 types of meat here, all of which are cooked beautifully. They also serve fish, including salmon, which they prepare in a unique fashion. And that's not all: They also have wonderful garnitures like mushrooms, green beans, salad and asparagus.

The interior of the restaurant, which is located on 44th Street, is mostly wooden. The waiters are also very experienced and American, so they speak English very well – which is important so that you can get their wonderful description of the food. Morton's also has a wide, affordable and decent wine menu. Last, the positioning of the tables also offers diners privacy, meaning you can have a nice chat with your friends, even if you're a large group.

NOBU DOWNTOWN

A huge chain with 30 branches around the world, Nobu serves up delectable Peruvian-Japanese fusion cuisine. The New York branch was Nobu's second following one in Los Angeles. Observing the place's success, the restaurant opened a second branch right next door called, appropriately enough, Nobu Next Door. In the end, what started as a simple Japanese restaurant has now spread around the world, offering the highest of quality from London to Cape Town.

Last year, however, Nobu closed down the NY Downtown and Next Door branches, opening a single new branch on the entrance floor of a historical building called Nobu Downtown. I only found out about the change by coincidence, but I sure did love it thanks to its high ceilings, spacious environment and thoughtful decoration. There's a bar and small tables at the entrance, as well as a sushi bar. They have a wide menu, although the menu on this floor is comparatively limited – that's not to say you won't enjoy your meal though!

The main restaurant is below. Personally, I didn't like this level too much because the ceilings were too low; it feels like a punishment to hang out in this place when there's such a wonderful atmosphere above. Besides, it's pretty hard to find a place, as it gets crowded between 5:30 and 7:30 p.m. since it's close to the business area. Perhaps the best idea is to spend an hour on the entrance floor and enjoy what's on the menu with a glass or two of good wine.

PER SE

Thomas Keller's French Laundry, a place with three Michelin stars, is as famous as himself. But when Keller wanted to open a restaurant in New York, Per Se was born. Located in Time Warner Plaza, Per Se has a superb view of Central Park – thanks in part to its one elevated area. Per Se has seating for 75 people, as well as tables that can sit a maximum of six people each.

Keller prepared the menu, although another chef cooks in the kitchen. It's open every evening, while it also serves lunch from Thursday to Sunday. Note that the menu isn't à la carte. Menu A, for instance, has 10 types of food from seafood to meat, while Menu B is prepared specifically with vegetarians in mind (both menus have the same price). Now Per Se is a pretty expensive place, but it's still hard to find reservations, so you might wish to opt for lunch, which is slightly cheaper.

RED ROOSTER

I've been going to this reasonably priced restaurant and bar in Harlem for the past 10 years to sample their New Orleans cuisine. I would suggest you go on Sunday at noon, or perhaps in the evening, when jazz groups from New Orleans take the stage. If you love listening to jazz and like dining as if you're having a snack, definitely take my advice! Nevertheless, you need to make a reservation. There's also a little terrace in front. My favorite thing at Red Rooster might just be the fried and sweet cornbread.

SUSHI OF GARI

There are three Sushi of Garis in New York, all of which I believe are wonderful. Nevertheless, I suggest that you head to the very first Sushi of Gari, in Northeast Manhattan. Founded by a Japanese chef named Gari, this authentic and reasonably priced restaurant is now a chain in which each branch can host 30-40 people.

I always like to eat at the sushi bar. After all, real Japanese sushi experts work at the counter before you, serving you as soon as they finish. And if you're lucky, you might even find Gari himself working in the kitchen as well. One of the major reasons why I love this place – besides the excellent sushi and sashimi – is the hot sushi designed by Gari himself. Now, this isn't something you would get away with in Japan: I once went to a good sushi restaurant in Japan and asked the chef if he could prepare something with avocado. His reply? An angry retort of "Go to America." But at Sushi of Gari, you can find many types of sushi prepared with avocado or different ingredients. The tuna nigiri with tomato sauce, for example, is bedazzling: The tuna is cold, the rice is warm and the tomato sauce is hot. Sushi of Gari serves up seven or eight types of hot nigiri. And if you like avocado like me, try Gari's salmon skin salad.

UNION SQUARE CAFE
Union Square Cafe used to be a small restaurant run by a woman chef. The reasonably priced café, which took its name from its own neighborhood, served from 11 a.m. to 11:30 p.m. with different menus for lunch and dinner. It also had a good and broad wine menu. And although it had low ceilings, I loved the place. Alas, it eventually closed. Fast-forward to February 2017, when I learned that it had reopened with the same name in the same neighborhood, but this time with an even better location: a corner building that has high ceilings, which pervades it with so much more light. Adding it up, it's the same menu and same chef, but with a stronger atmosphere.

It's often impossible to find a place at this restaurant, but you might be in luck at about 3:30 p.m. Although the menu at this hour is limited, you'll still find some delicious food. You can also try the same menu at the bar, where you don't require a reservation (you can work your way through the whole menu if you go a couple of times). What's more, their service is great.

NICE

THE BEST TIME TO VISIT THE SOUTH OF FRANCE: SUMMER

The south of France is a dreamy coastal strip with breathtaking towns and beautiful cities. Whether to the east or west of Nice, there are incredible views, delicious restaurants and impressive hotels. That being said, I have a couple of recommendations for your next trip to Nice.

Nice and its vicinity are great at the beginning of summer. Here, the French Riviera consists of intriguing small towns and villages right up to the Italian border. But don't let the word village fool you: Rich families from both France and elsewhere spend an amazing time in these villages for a couple of months every year. Nice is a truly unforgettable destination thanks to its turquoise blue sea, sandy beaches, elegant streets, delicious food and vibrant nightlife, so make sure you start your French Riviera tour from there.

If you're coming from Istanbul, it's easy to get to Nice; many airlines have two or three flights per day between the two cities. Paris might be 3.5 hours from Istanbul, but Nice is just 2.5 hours, making it a shorter and easier flight. And with the city on the Mediterranean, the cold weather of northern France is nowhere to be found here. And, as I noted above, there's beauty all around the area: Head out 50 km in either direction from Nice's airport and you're bound to find somewhere beautiful. The only downside is there's just not enough time to time to truly experience every single town on the French Riviera, but if you can, do try and take in Cap Ferrat, Villefrenche, Monaco, Menton, Saint-Paul-de-Vence, Grasse, Antibes and Cannes.

My favorite restaurant in Nice is La Petite Maison. Foodies will know, it's an amazing restaurant and has a branch in Istanbul as well. It has become a franchise, with branches in London, Abu Dhabi, Dubai, Miami, Hong Kong and Istanbul, but the branch in Nice is the original. The passionate Madame Nicole first opened La Petite Maison, but she now runs it with her daughter and sister. I've had the chance to go to a few La Petite Maisons around the world; they're all nice, but the one in Nice is something else, especially as Madame Nicole's presence in the restaurant creates a different kind of spirit. Another good aspect of the restaurant is that they have live music on Friday and Saturday nights from 10:30 p.m. to midnight. Thankfully, though, it's not noisy or disturbing at all. There are no mics and no speakers – just a couple of musicians making music in between the tables. Whatever you do, take some time to dine at La Petite Maison when you're in Nice. And if you're going there for lunch, you can enjoy the terrace (the terrace is also a good choice for dinner on warm summer nights).

HEADING TOWARD MONACO

Head out east from Nice and you'll soon come to Cap Ferrat, where my favorite hotel is La Voile d'Or, a small place by the sea. Now, most beaches in the area are public, but La Voile d'Or's visitors can get exclusive access to the hotel's beach, meaning it's never that crowded. And because the wind typically blows from the coast to the sea, the water is always brilliant. The hotel's restaurant, meanwhile, is also a favorite of mine.

Along the coastal strip, Villefrenche-sur-Mer comes after Cap Ferrat. Villefrenche is a stunningly beautiful village with an amazing coastline and numerous restaurants. In fact, Villefrenche is a modern fishing village, meaning the Côte d'Azur's best fish are in town. My favorite restaurant here is La Mère Germain (est. 1938), which has delicious food and wonderful service. Run by the founding family's fourth generation, La Mère Germain is growing day by day – by the time they reach their centennial in 2038, they might have taken up the whole coastline. While La Mère Germain is always full of people waiting to get in, the neighboring restaurants are mostly empty. The establishment owes this success to its two bosses, who happen to be brothers as well. At La Mère Germain, they do all the jobs without letting their egos get in the way.

After Villefrenche-sur-Mer, our next stop is the Principality of Monaco. It's a small country, but you can also think of it as a large company with a king as its CEO. Invest in a good real estate opportunity and say goodbye to income tax with a Monaco passport – a great way to head to Europe or the U.S. with ease if your present passport doesn't afford you such opportunity.

It's no surprise that there are many restaurants in this grandiose country. You're spoiled for choice, but the best one is Hôtel de Paris, which boasts more than a few stars. Alain Ducasse is on the scene with his restaurant, Le Louis XV, for those willing to part with a pretty penny by the end of the night. You even have a chance to see the great man himself often at this restaurant, as well as the newest dishes and the oldest tasting menu. If you want to come here and pay "less," the place is also open at noon. But if you're not in the habit of spending money at a three-starred restaurant, Café de Paris right across from Le Louis XV offers good fare for a tenth of the cost. Just don't order Café de Paris steak, because there isn't any! They removed it from the menu a long time ago, but apparently the news hasn't traveled far, because there's always at least one person at every table that wants to order it. As for me, I can't really fathom why they don't include such a popular dish on their menu. And here's another useful tip for Monaco: carry your passport with you if you want to cheer up with a little bit of wine and fun at the casino. Otherwise, you won't be able to play.

LA TURBIE/HOSTELLERIE JEROME

La Turbie is a very small beautiful village uphill from the coast. There is the famous little hotel there with an extraordinary restaurant: Hostellerie Jerome. You should either visit La Turbie for a few hours and have lunch at Jerome and go back. But be careful with the wine as the wine list is extraordinary and tempting. Or go there for dinner and indulge yourself to the wine list with the extraordinary food and sleep at the hotel after dinner. Next morning enjoy a Michelin star breakfast at the hotel or a smaller one at one of the beautiful cafes of the village square. You will be happy either way to enjoy some countryside silence after the buzz of Cote d'Azur.

MENTON

The last stop before Italy is Menton, the home of the world's best restaurants, Mirazur. Heading up the restaurant is an Argentine chef who cooks French dishes. If you want ironed cotton tablecloth like me, they'll immediately bring one to you. If you don't, you'll be eating at a wooden table as if you're at a kebab place. And given the location, you won't be surprised to hear that it has an unreal view.

San Remo is really close to Menton, but I don't have any specific restaurant recommendations for there. But if you've ever watched the San Remo Music Festival that used be aired on TV, you might want to stop by for a trip down memory lane.

ANTIBES

Back in the other direction, to the west of Nice, is Antibes. Le Figuier du Saint Esprit is a restaurant managed by Christian Morisset, a mustachioed famous chef who has worked in two or three Michelin-starred restaurants along the Côte d'Azure. After Morisset decided to start his own business two years ago, he established this restaurant in a village called Saint Esprit, serving up delicious French meals and high-quality wine. Morisset himself is in the kitchen, while his wife organizes the service. And to allow diners to know what is happening in the kitchen, he put up a big-screen television on the wall for the customers. There's so much going on in the kitchen come rush hour that you'll hardly talk to those at your table. Consciously, though, he decided to keep this place at a single star, although that obviously doesn't mean it's short on any quality.

The restaurant was built around a fig tree located in the very middle – the very fig tree after which the restaurant is named (and from which you can still eat, if you so desire). French restaurants are generally closed on Sundays and Mondays, but Christian Morisset opens on those days, closing only on Tuesdays. Though perhaps less well-known than other places along the French Riviera, Le Figuier du Saint Esprit is certainly worth a trip thanks to its delicious food and great atmosphere.

CANNES

Head further west and you'll get closer to Cannes, but before you do, take a pit stop at Josy Jo in Haute de Cagnes, which is run by a septuagenarian in a 300-year-old building. It's a busy place that features about 40 workers. It's also somewhere that you should book ahead of time to guarantee a table.

Back on the road, it's time to head to Cannes – the summer playground for the rich. Come Easter, houses that sit empty for six months of the year start to fill up once more. And by July or August, it's nearly impossible to walk on the street. It's also so crowded that the beaches are full, regardless of the time of day, meaning that if your hotel's own private beach is full, there will most certainly be no room at the public beach. The best time to come here, accordingly, is in September and October. By fall, however, the restaurants have become more spoiled and the waiters more than a little tired. I reckon the best time to come is at the beginning of June, right after the Cannes Film Festival. More than that, you can even see that Turkish is competing with Russian in its quest to become the second language on the streets of Cannes if you wait for school to end before coming.

My favorite restaurant in Cannes is Le Park 45, which has one Michelin star at a location somewhat removed from the street noise. Le Park 45 also has a head waiter who is French but who spent his childhood in Istanbul, so you'll love hearing him speak Turkish if you happen to know it. And best of all, if you have a good wine with you, bring it along, as you'll only have to pay a small corkage fee.

And while you're in Cannes, make sure you have a few snacks and a glass of wine on the terrace of the Carlton in the afternoon.

SAINT-PAUL-DE-VENCE

Continuing a bit more to the west toward the mountains, we arrive at Saint-Paul-de-Vence to eat at Colombe d'Or.

Tables with white tablecloths in the garden are at your service when the weather's nice. But it's not a problem if it starts to rain while you're eating, as there are tables available inside as well.

In Saint-Paul-de-Vence there is a hotel called Château Saint Martin. Beautiful and expensive, it's not a place that you need to stay in, but it is a must in terms of lunch or dinner. For me, it's a place imbued with special meaning, as I celebrated my 40th birthday in this hotel, as well as my 60th. If all goes well, I hope to celebrate my 80th here as well, and maybe even my 100th!

A SUNDAY STROLL IN NICE

If you're in Nice on a Sunday, definitely visit a marketplace. Skip the hotel breakfast and head for Vieux Nice, the old center where the town was formed a thousand years ago. Covered with stone buildings, there's a big marketplace in the middle of buildings. The market is open seven days a week, but Sunday is the big day, when farmers from nearby villages sell their fresh products, from eggs to tomatoes, mushrooms and cheese. The market opens at 8 a.m. and closes at 1 p.m., as there's nothing left by that time. Coincidentally, all Nice-Istanbul flights are after 1 p.m., so you could, theoretically, do your weekly grocery shopping in Vieux Nice, hop on a plane back to Istanbul and enjoy fresh ingredients from the Riviera all week long. I prefer to buy cheese, zucchini blossoms, baby asparagus and mushrooms, as their prices aren't that different from what I buy in Istanbul. I usually take an empty suitcase with me, fill it with food and bring back to Istanbul.

Cafes and restaurants also abound the marketplace, so you can dig into breakfast in one of them after a bout of shopping (although I myself prefer to pick up food and eat as I stroll the market before hitting up a cafe for coffee or tea). Whatever the case, I can't imagine being in Nice on a Sunday and not going there.

SOCCA, THE STAR OF THE VIEUX NICE MARKET

One of the most enjoyable things to do while you're strolling the market is to eat Socca cooked by a middle-aged lady in the market. Socca is a type of pancake made with olive oil and chickpea flour. First, you turn the dough into a liquid and then pour it into an iron plate in a thin layer. After cooking it, you take it out, put it into a roll and serve.

PIZZA FROM NICE: PISSALADIÈRE

The specialty pizza from Nice has but olive oil in its dough, along with a fried onion on top – there are no other ingredients involved. It's actually a delicious food for the poor. When in Nice, definitely try a piece of this vegetarian pizza.

OSAKA

Tokyo has pride of place in Japan, but the most important cities after the capital are Osaka and Kyoto. For people from Turkey, it's never been easier to get to Osaka, as Turkish Airlines now flies there direct.

We hit up Osaka, staying in the Imperial Hotel to get a feel for both it and Kyoto. The hotel includes a sushi restaurant, a classic Japanese restaurant, as well as a Chinese restaurant – all of which are good options if you want to grab a bite on the go.

No sooner had we landed in Osaka than we headed to a typical Japanese restaurant called Taian. The sushi was good, as were the other Japanese meals on the menu. Taian only has seating for 20: 10 at the sushi bar and 10 at the tables. Hard at work behind the sushi bar are four or five sushi chefs who, if you're lucky, will occasionally give you a few small treats if you're sitting right by them.

Now, the tradition at a Japanese restaurant is as follows: When you call for a reservation, they immediately tell you about the price of their menus, and you choose your preference right at that moment. At the same time, you also indicate the ingredients that you won't eat. Thanks to this, your menu is ready when you arrive at the restaurant! What's more, everything is prepared right in front of you. And when you ask for the wine menu, they'll just ask you to choose between white and red; now, you might think that they have separate menus for white and red, but you'll soon realize that there are just two types of wine – no lists, no menus, just two types of wine. This is mostly the case everywhere – even in three-star restaurants. Thankfully, however, Taian had a decent wine list, which meant we had a wonderful meal with wine.

While at Taian, we started to chat with a retired Japanese surgeon at the next table. The restaurant we had lined up for the day after was really far away and, to be honest, I wasn't eager on going there. I duly asked for some restaurant advice from this gentleman, who now spends his days enjoying his retirement with his wife. I wanted a nice, normal place that the locals enjoyed – something without a Michelin star. He gave us a card with the address, in Japanese, of one of his favorite restaurants. Thanks to the efforts of a cab driver, we were able to reach the restaurant, a sushi place with room for a maximum of 15 people. They didn't ask about our menu choices beforehand like most places do, but they did ask us for our preferences. My daughter and I plumped for different choices of sushi, which they prepared wonderfully. It was only later that I learned the place's name: Dojima and Human.

PARIS

French cuisine is renowned for being the best in the world, so it's no surprise that food is an art form in Paris. Sampling amazing dishes in the magical atmosphere of the City of Love is definitely a privilege. I travel a lot to Paris for business, meaning I'm lucky enough to try new restaurants every time. Inevitably, there's another marvelous restaurant to add to my recommendation list with every passing day...

I've previously written about Paris' restaurants, but I reckon it's time for an update, since I've tried many new restaurants in the intervening time and I've realized that some of the places I went to before aren't all they're cracked up to be. And as you all know, once is never enough for a city like Paris.

Below I've listed 10 Parisian restaurants in alphabetical order. Some of these places boast three Michelin stars, and some have none, but all of them will surely leave you feeling more than satisfied. If you're in the French capital, definitely make your way to as many of these places as you can.

ANTOINE
(10 Avenue de New York, 75116 Paris Tel: 33 1 40 70 19 28)
Antoine, a restaurant with one Michelin star, is located near the Seine River, right in front of the Eiffel Tower. A young chef runs the place, which is heavy on fish and other seafood. The place is open for lunch (when prices are better) and dinner. Many restaurants in Paris don't have a lot of windows, making you focus on the food alone. But with Antoine so close to the Eiffel

Tower, it's no wonder that the restaurant has big windows, because it's got the best view of the famous landmark in town. In the end, Antoine is a place that offers the perfect trio of view, food and wine.

APICIUS
(20, Rue d'Artais, 75008 Paris   Tel: 33 1 43 80 19 66)

Apicius, a place I've mentioned before, is a restaurant owned by a 50-year-old chef, Jean-Pierre Vigato. It's located in a grand historical villa in a garden, meaning the restaurant is very spacious – to the degree that you almost forget that you're in a metropolis. The reason Apicius is on my list is their excellent tasting menu. Sometimes, they have two tasting menus, although you can make changes if there is a dish that you don't fancy in the menu you choose. Apicius has an extensive wine menu and, even better, its prices aren't even that high. Apicius is, however, slowly becoming more popular, making it harder to arrange reservations. This increasing popularity is naturally reflected in their prices, but apart from this, the food is great!

Apicius has a charming terrace used in the summer. They don't serve dinner on the terrace, although you can have drinks there before your meal. Back in the day, Apicius' lunch used to be cheaper, but now that it's hard to make reservations for either lunch or dinner, the lunch menu's price is the same as the dinner menu. Still, if you're willing to shell out a little bit for good food, then Apicius is a nice option.

ÉPICURE

(Le Bristol, 112 Rue du Faubourg Saint-Honoré, 75008 Paris   Tel: 33 1 53 43 43 40)

Épicure, located in Le Bristol Hotel, is a Paris restaurant I truly love. There are many "palaces" in Paris, but Le Bristol is the only hotel located in one of these buildings. The hotel has a very pretty yard, but unlike some hotels, Épicure doesn't cover the top to create a winter garden, meaning you can eat outside when the weather is good. The restaurant accommodates up to 40 customers, seven days a week, for lunch and dinner (unlike most Parisian restaurants with two or three stars that usually stay closed on Saturdays and Sundays). A comfortable place, Épicure has great service and a very good wine menu. They even have three different sommeliers on hand to help you choose your wine.

As for the menu, Épicure has a number of dishes with fish and vegetables, while I really appreciated that they have white truffles on the menu as well (come fall, you can also find black truffles from Perigord). The place isn't very crowded at noon, so the prices are better at that time of day. The menu might be more limited at that time, but you still get the same service and the food is still amazingly good.

ITINÉRAIRES

(5 Rue de Pontoise, 75005 Paris   Tel: 33 1 46 33 60 11)

Located in Saint-Germain, this inviting, one-star restaurant is run by a husband-and-wife team, with the man in the kitchen and the woman serving. One of the things I like the most about this 40-person restaurant is their bread; as soon as you sit down, they bring you fresh bread. Moreover, they bring you a French baguette right out of the oven with your dish. No matter when you arrive, the customers are always greeted with fresh bread. When you think about it, this is actually something very hard to accomplish, yet they've somehow managed to pull it off. But this nuance in the service is really significant for someone like me: I really love to eat good bread. They also bring delicious, homemade chocolates and cookies with your coffee.

I think the food is fantastic – so much so that I asked the chef why they still hadn't scored a second Michelin star. Interestingly enough, he said: "I don't want to get a second Michelin star on purpose. If we have another star, new expenses will appear, the cost of the dishes will increase and ultimately, we'll be too expensive for our customers. We want this place to be full all the time." Given that, it's clear that Itinéraires is the best place to eat a two-star meal for the price of one!

LE PUR
(Park Hyatt Paris 5, Rue de La Paix, 75002 Paris   Tel: 33 1 58 71 12 34)
Le Pur is located in the Park Hyatt Hotel. A place with one Michelin star, Le Put only serves dinner and not on Sundays. Jean François Rouquette is the young chef of the place. They prepare light dishes for a very large menu. Naturally, the dishes are fairly simple and, accordingly, reasonably priced. They also have some nice things for appetizers.

On my previous visit to Le Pur, I couldn't

decide whether the wine list was good or bad. There are, however, now two sommelières at Le Pur who are great at matching wines and informing diners about what's on offer. For instance, I went to Le Pur with a guest of mine; at the time, neither of us fancied any meat, so we asked to switch the dishes to fish. That, of course, necessitated a change in wine, but the sommelières had no problem immediately changing our wines. While there, I tried wines I had never tasted before, and I liked all of them.

MONSIEUR BLEU
(20 Avenue de New York, 75116 Paris   Tel: 33 1 47 20 90 47)
Monsieur Bleu is a restaurant that bears a lot of resemblance to 29 or Sunset in Turkey, even if it is a bit larger than them. Monsieur Bleu is a place for every age, thanks in part to a huge bar, nice music in the background, as well as a beautiful view of the Eiffel Tower (which puts it close to Antoine). But even in spite of the latter, the prices are still reasonable.

The best part about Monsieur Bleu is that you can dine outside in the summer and sample almost any food that you desire. They serve in two sessions: the first one at 7:30 p.m. and the second at 9:30 p.m. If you're up for eating quickly and then leaving, then make reservations for 7:30, but if you want to continue at the bar, you should choose the second session. As the night continues, the place turns into a bit of a nightclub, drawing in the chic and the famous with its vibrancy and live music (which is in contrast to other upper-crust French restaurants). I took my daughter and her friends to the second session; they loved

Monsieur Bleu so much that we stayed there for hours, and there's a good chance they wouldn't have enjoyed the other restaurants I mentioned as much as they enjoyed Monsieur Bleu. All in all, it's a restaurant that's sure to please you.

NAKATANI
(27 rue Pierre Leroux 75007 Paris   Tel: 01 47 34 94 14)
Nakatani gets its name from its Japanese chef, and like many Japanese restaurants, it has minimalist decoration. But make no mistake, this is a French restaurant through and through, even if there are occasional Japanese flourishes in the meal (the chef himself grew up in France). There are two different menus with similar prices. Beware, though, that they do not serve à la carte, so you have to choose which menu you're going to eat. I chose the menu with the seafood, and I had no regrets. One drawback, however, is Nakatani's location, which is a 20-minute drive from the city center.

NEIGE D'ÉTÉ
(12, rue de l'Amiral Roussin, 75015 Paris   Tel: 33 1 42 73 66 66)
Neige d'été is a small French restaurant with one Michelin star. It has room for just 30 people, in part because they have a huge open kitchen that takes up a third of the space. For a second, you feel like you're eating in the kitchen, but Neige d'été's ventilation is so good that the smell of the food in the kitchen doesn't bother you. One of the great things about this place is they serve wine by the glass, but more than that, they

also let you have a full or half glass – something that is rare indeed. Thus, you can try as many wines as you'd like to. Moreover, they write the wines they're serving on a blackboard. All in all, Neige d'été gets a thumbs up from me thanks to its simplicity and reasonable prices.

TAILLEVENT
(15 Rue Lamennais, 75008 Paris   Tel: 33 1 44 95 15 01)

One of the oldest and most expensive restaurants in Paris, Taillevent is a place best avoided in the evening because the prices are sky high. And when the food is that expensive, you'll inevitably pay a fortune for wine as well. Intriguingly, though, Taillevent is quite empty at noon for some reason, meaning they serve far more reasonably priced menus at that time of day. So, if you want to try Taillevent, look at the days they're open and make some early reservations for lunchtime. They also have a large wine list.

ZE KITCHEN
(4 Rue des Grands Augustins, 75006 Paris   Tel: 33 1 44 32 00 32)

Ze Kitchen, which can accommodate 30-40 people, is best described as a place that cooks fusion dishes, with two-thirds of the dishes French and the remainder Japanese. You can either visit Ze Kitchen for lunch or dinner – the prices for both are quite reasonable. The service is also pretty good, although the wine menu leaves a bit to be desired.

CULINARY TOURISM

Restaurants with three stars in Paris generally host no more than 50 people and are usually closed two days a week. Tourists who are willing to shell out a lot of cash while traveling generally check the Michelin Guide for a good restaurant to eat (there are 10 restaurants with three stars). Such tourists then ask the concierge of their hotel to make a reservation for one of the restaurants. With so many people coming to these restaurants in such a fashion, it's no wonder that these kinds of tourists constitute the main customer group of these fine-dining establishments. Occasionally, terrorist attacks or economic crises will create a brief dip in terms of popularity, but never for very long. These restaurants have such an ambience, quality and service that rich tourists won't abstain from paying a fortune for a course for very long. I reckon this is also one of the reasons behind the skyrocketing prices of three-starred restaurants in Paris.

WHY IS A LARGE WINE MENU GOOD?

Having a large wine list has some advantages. If you're a knowledgeable wine person, you can make your choice easily. But even if you are, you might also want to learn something from the sommelier of the place. For instance, you might want to taste a wine that you don't know but, at the same time, you don't want to pay too much either; in such a case, your salvation lies with the sommelier. To be successful, I believe you need a cellar of at least a thousand types of wines. That's hard to do in Turkey, but in Paris, places with a decent wine menu have at least 2,000 types of wine. In the end, these kinds of wine cellars might be worth more than the place itself.

5 ENJOYABLE –AND REASONABLY PRICED – RESTAURANTS IN PARIS:

Hollybelly
Breakfast and brunch
No reservations
19 rue Lucien Sampaix, 75010

Huitrerie Régis
Oysters
No reservations
3 rue de Montfaucon, 75006

Mamma Primi
Italian
No reservations
71 rue des Dames, 75017

L'assiette aux fromages
Fondue
Raclette
25 rue Mouffetard, 75005

Chez Michel
Countryside French & terrific deserts
10 rue de Belzunce, 75010

RIO

Rio de Janeiro is one of the most enticing destinations in South America; it's also the city that has stolen my heart again after 20 years. But with its beautiful beaches, friendly people and surprising restaurants, I'm sure it would steal your heart too.

Compared to before, it's now much easier to travel to Rio, as Turkish Airlines has a direct flight from Istanbul to São Paulo every day, allowing you to arrive in Rio by the evening. By that time, the best thing to do is to have a light dinner and get to sleep after a 14-hour flight. When you wake up the next day, shake off the jet lag with a bit of a swim in the sea. Rio obviously never gets particularly cold, but it's probably best to go there between November and March.

When I first went to Rio two decades ago, the place had a lot of economic problems, like inflation and currency devaluation, that also fomented chaos on the streets. Everyone warned us to be careful while walking outside; we took the advice to heart and generally steered clear of the streets.

Years later, I decided to go to Rio with my daughter; as we were planning to go, however, I learned that one of my university friends had since moved there, settling down after marrying a Brazilian woman. Now the owner of a tourism agency, he related his lovely story of how he ended up in Brazil.

YOU COME AND YOU NEVER WANT TO LEAVE

My friend told his family that he wanted to go on holiday to South America after graduation. His family gave his assent and off he went. But when the time came to return, he found he just couldn't.

"A couple of weeks aren't enough for Brazil, and besides, this place is really cheap," he said to himself. "I could stay here another month with the money you gave me."

My friend duly asked for a bit more time from his family. But when the time came to leave again, he again found that he just couldn't bring himself to return. This time, he decided to stay for good. He eventually got married and established his own business.

He also explained the "danger" of staying too long: "If you stay here for a week, you end up deciding to come here again. If you stay here for two weeks, you'll come here every year. And if you stay here for three weeks, you never go back again."

Truer words have never been spoken!

It was wonderful to go back to Rio after 20 years. Everything has changed: You can safely walk in the streets, and the people are cheerful and more prosperous. At the hotel, they told us to avoid walking in the street with our mobile phones in our hands, but I couldn't see anyone on the street without a phone in their hand.

Despite the long flight, Rio de Janeiro has enchanted me once again, meaning I'm sure to return once again.

Ultimately, we headed to Rio in February, which allowed us to enjoy the 35-degree weather, the sea and, of course, some delicious meals. Thanks to our summer holiday, we managed to arrive back in the Northern Hemisphere fresh for spring!

One of the most beautiful things of Rio is, of course, the food and the restaurants. So allow me to run the rule over 10 restaurant and two hotels in Rio – organized, as always, alphabetically. And if you happen to visit them yourself, don't hesitate to drop a line.

CIPRIANI

Rio boasts two luxury hotels, one of which is the Copacabana Palace, which is located in a historical building across from the famous beach of the same name. The hotel's restaurant, meanwhile, is the Cipriani, which is like a lot of Ciprianis around the world. The restaurant, which can sit between 80 and 100, serves Italian cuisine that uses local fresh vegetables and fish. People generally want to have meat when they go to Brazil, but eating vegetables, fish or pasta is another good option. But while the fare is good, Cipriani's wine selection is fairly limited. Still, if you're staying at the Copacabana, I highly recommend you give the Cipriani a try. But even if you're not staying at the hotel, this is still a great chance to dine at a beautiful restaurant.

CT BOUCHERIE

CT Boucherie is a French restaurant that predominantly serves meat from the grill. They serve their meat with plenty of garnish, while there are also salads on the menu. At the same time, they can also serve you fish if you're not up for meat. The portions in Brazil are generally big, albeit not at CT Boucherie – but that means that this place is a good option for a light lunch.

ESPLANADA GRILL

Esplanada Grill is surrounded by a number of fancy boutiques, offering you a chance to people-watch as the more elegant of Rio's women stop by for a break after a bout of shopping. Intent on not gaining weight, most of these women opt merely for some salad and water, but there's no stopping the assorted businessmen at the grill from digging into meat and fresh fish. Esplanada also has great garnitures and pasta.

THE BEST THREE PLACES

Because of the Brazilian population's multicultural roots, it's possible to find European traces in the country's cuisine. One thing that was really surprising to me, however, was Brazilians' ability to endlessly pack away so much meat and fish. In truth, you hardly enjoy the taste of food after you get full, yet they're used to – and, indeed, enjoy – consuming vast quantities of meat and fish at a late hour. If you want to go all the restaurants that I've listed here, you'd need to stay in Rio at least a week. If you have far less time, at least make your way to Satyricon, Esplanada and Rio de Canerio.

FASANO

The Fasano is the best hotel in Ipanema. The place also has a lovely fish restaurant that serves small-portioned dishes and pasta for both lunch and dinner. Fasano has a separate bar, which helps give it a bit of the atmosphere of a nightclub.

Now, they might be used to big portions of meat in South America, but as tourists, it's probably best to skip such a huge smorgasbord. If you have a big lunch, it's probably better to go light on dinner or vice versa (especially as they have their evening meals at 11 p.m., a time when I'm usually getting ready to sleep). Lunches, accordingly, are a far more suitable alternative, starting at 2 p.m. and continuing on until 5. You can get your daily amount of calories between these hours, allowing you to skip a big dinner in favor of a light bite instead.

FOGO DE CHÃO
Fogo de Chão is a famous meat restaurant in Rio. It truly is a paradise for meat lovers! When you sit down, they give you a card, with one red side and one green side. As long as you leave the green side up, they will continue to serve you meat; when you can ingest no more, you flip the card over to the red side. There are 10 different kinds of meat at Fogo de Chão, with different waiters serving different kinds of meat. Every waiter cooks and serves the meat that he or she is in charge of. And if you still have room after all that meat, you can choose from a broad dessert menu. My advice to you: If you can't resist the temptation for meat at Fogo de Chão, make sure your next meals are lighter!

MARIUS
Marius is a famous restaurant in Rio that, like Fogo de Chão, also uses the green/red-card system. Instead of meat, however, they will keep serving you a vast array of fish and seafood until you flip your card to the red side. Marius has a wide-ranging dessert menu as well. The price for a meat-based meal at Marius is about 200

TL, while it's about 300 TL for a fish meal, although wine is not included, so the cost may be a bit higher depending on the quality of the wine you choose.

PORÇÃO

A very popular restaurant, Porção serves both meat and fish. They ask you what you would like to eat first, then they serve you until you give up and flip the card to red. Porção has a wide range of salads and garnitures – so much that you can satisfy yourself just by having salad. It also serves a wide array of desserts.

SATYRICON

The fish restaurant Satyricon is my favorite restaurant in Rio. The restaurant's system took me back to my childhood and Urcan Restaurant in Sarıyer, where you would choose a fresh fish for your meal before enjoying a green salad as you waited for your meal. (They do the same thing now in Yalıkavak in Bodrum.) When a group of four of us went to Satyricon, we chose a big fish that was big enough for six people, along with a crayfish for each of us. Before the fish came, we enjoyed a salad, as well as a few starters. Then came the special part: the fish, served as a whole. We topped everything off with a dessert. But perhaps the best part about Satyricon is its broad wine menu; as for us, we chose a good Chilean wine, even ordering a second bottle.

RIO DE CENARIO

Rio de Cenario is actually a dance studio, meaning music and dance provides an accompanying soundtrack at this restaurant, which is located inside a century-old, high-ceilinged building. An orchestra featuring a group of eight to ten, including two women soloists, takes the stage between 9 and 11 p.m. You can wile away the night dancing in a wonderful historical building; we, for one, had hours of enjoyment in the company of French champagne.

SUDBRACK

Sudbrack is a boutique fusion restaurant that was established by 45-year-old Roberta Sudbrack, a person who evidently enjoys cooking. Sudbrack has worked in top restaurants overseas; upon her return to Brazil, she applied the techniques she learned to Brazilian cuisine.

The restaurant seats 40 people on two stories, while there are 10 staff, most of whom are women, who work in the kitchen on the top floor.

Sudbrack brings six or seven different portions from its gastronomical menu. While there, my daughter and I went for fish. If they ever get around to awarding a Michelin star to a Brazilian restaurant, Sudbrack will be the first to get it.

The prices might be a bit on the high side, but the wine selection is remarkable. Note, however, that the place isn't really suited for lunch as it's usually quite empty at that time.

IPANEMA: THE HEART OF ENTERTAINMENT

There are two popular beaches in Rio de Janeiro, Copacabana and Ipanema. The latter is the site of many expensive hotels and luxurious boutiques, as well as home to some colorful nightlife. The area itself, however, is peaceful, so you will see people enjoying the beach everywhere.

ROME

ARCHIMEDE: A REAL, POPULAR RESTAURANT

Located on the Piazza dei Caprettari, Archimede is a real, popular and family-run restaurant that serves up Italian cuisine, largely for Romans, rather than tourists. Now 80 years old, Archimede is now in the hands of the third generation. Open for lunch and dinner, Archimede also has both indoor and outdoor seating.

They have a wide antipasto buffet that consists of salads and vegetables cooked and fried with olive oil. You can start by preparing an antipasto plate for yourself before moving on to one of their 15 types of traditional Italian pasta, if you wish. A particular hit is the pasta with lobster. Although lobster is generally a pricey food, it's quite affordable at Archimede, costing only about 20 euros. Mind you, if you go to Rome in October or November, you might also want to try the pasta with porcini mushrooms, which will be in season.

They also serve daily fresh fish, but it's always best to ask for the fish of the day before ordering. And after the main course, there's a little buffet with desserts and fruits.

Archimede's portions are quite big, so I suggest you only go for the main course. For myself, I chose a menu consisting of antipasto, pasta and fresh fruit. If you go there at lunch, make sure to sit outside and enjoy the view of the piazza.

Expect to pay approximately 40 or 50 euros for your entire meal.

DAL BOLOGNESE:
TYPICAL ITALIAN FARE

The second cheapest restaurant on the list, Dal Bolognese has been serving up typical Italian fare on Piazza del Poppolo for almost 70 or 80 years. You can eat inside, but it's better to go outside when the weather is nice. And come October, November or December, the smell of white truffles pervades Dal Bolognese, but if you go at any other time, it's not possible to find the delicious fungi (as is the case with porcini mushrooms). Whatever you do, give these mushrooms a try if you go right in season.

Like many other Italian restaurants, the seats are a bit crowded, so you might have difficulty talking to the rest of your company. If you keep the wine intake down, a meal at Dal Bolognese will probably set you back about 60 or 70 euros. Reservations, meanwhile, are not required for lunch.

LE JARDIN DE RUSSIE:
JOY IN THE GARDEN

I'm not talking about hotels today, but I can't help but mention Hotel de Russie, one of my favorite hotels in the Eternal City. Hotel de Russie belongs to Rocco Forte, a brand of a British hotel group. Like the others in the chain, it is a boutique hotel. More than that, it's the best place for accommodation in Rome. The building is surrounded by a courtyard or, you could say, a big, layered garden. There is a bar on the ground floor of the garden, while the top floor is used as a restaurant called Le Jardin de Russie.

Rome's weather is nice six months of the year, so it's a real treat to enjoy a drink outside in the garden come summer. The restaurant has a 60-person capacity, while the accompanying café has a 100-person capacity. The place, run by Fulvio Pierangelini, is a hit with both locals and tourists for lunch and dinner. (Lunch, you will guess, would be absolutely perfect in the garden in summer.) Le Jardin de Russie serves traditional Italian food alongside a wide-ranging wine menu for an affordable price. Even if I don't stay in the Hotel de Russie, I also come to the restaurant for a meal. A meal here will set you back about 80 or 90 euros.

LA PERGOLA: ROME'S ONLY THREE-STAR RESTAURANT

Our last restaurant is La Pergola, which is well-known by tourists. For me, it is the best restaurant in the Italian capital. The restaurant is located near the Vatican, inside the Waldorf Astoria Cavalieri Hotel. Le Pergola, which has a German chef named Heinz Beck, is the only restaurant in Rome with three Michelin stars, meaning it typically draws rich tourists. Given such elegance, it's no surprise that you should try to make a reservation a couple of months ahead of time.

You can enjoy traditional Italian dishes at this magnificent restaurant, but why don't you experience Beck's special gastronomical menu for 200 euros, excluding wine. But whatever you eat, the food is delicious, especially the gnocchi and cheese.

Le Pergola is open every day except Sunday and Monday, while it also closes its doors in January and August.

The restaurant's wine cellar is also bursting at the seams, with 50,000 different types of wines, making it one of the biggest in the country alongside Enoteca Pinchiorri in Florence. This means that you'll need to spend a long time choosing a wine, although you can download the wine list ahead of time to help you make a decision.

SAN SEBASTIAN

Spain has taken great strides to become a center of gastronomy over the past decade. More than a few of the country's eating establishments have risen to become some of the world's most important restaurants, including El Bulli, which I've mentioned on previous occasions.

Some of these restaurants serve surprising and extraordinary dishes, while others offer more typical Spanish fare. Still others might serve just Catalan or classic Basque dishes. Both of these regions are located not far from France: From El Bulli in Catalonia in the northeast of Spain, it's just a 30-minute drive to France. Likewise, from San Sebastian in the Basque Country in the country's north, it's just a half-hour drive to the French border. But while you might think that you see French traces in Spanish cuisine, you would be wrong, especially in the case of Catalan cuisine, which has no French traces.

If you're coming from Turkey, Turkish Airlines flies directly to Bilbao, from where it's just a hop, skip and a jump of one hour to San Sebastian.

WHERE TO STAY IN SAN SEBASTIAN?
In San Sebastian, I stayed in the Maria Christina Hotel – a place I highly recommend. It's in the perfect location for guests who want to walk or swim. The only drawback? It only has a subpar Chinese restaurant (given the plethora of Michelin-starred restaurants in the vicinity, I assume they wanted to create an alternative). Still, the breakfast is nice.

Sporting a classical interior design, the Marina

Christina is located in an old building, although it has been newly refurbished and restored.

I stayed in Bilbao just one night, but I did not like my hotel, so if you come across any possibility, please do keep me informed. That aside, the Guggenheim Museum in Bilbao is a magnificent place; if anything, the exterior is even more breathtaking than the artwork inside. The museum is almost worthy of extending your trip to see.

MYRIADS OF STARRED RESTAURANTS

Because some high-end restaurants are often closed on Mondays, if not Sundays, I specifically chose Friday and Saturday to visit (although some places are open on Sundays for lunch). Now, in an effort to eat everywhere, you may think you can visit up to five or six restaurants in just two days by just eating light, but you really can't: Sometimes it takes three or more hours to actually try a restaurant's menu. That's why it's better to just go for a light lunch and then try the menus for dinner so that you get the full experience of the restaurant – even if that means trying fewer establishments.

San Sebastian has three three-star restaurants, as well as some two-star restaurants. In fact, there was one two-star restaurant I really wanted to visit, but the lack of time put paid to that, so it's on the list for next summer.

But at the risk of raising your ire, I'm not going to mention the best restaurant in San Sebastian. That's because I want people who visit these restaurants to make their own list. So let me share my opinions about three of the city's restaurants and then let me know based on your own opinions; that'll allow us to compare!

San Sebastian gets more than its share of rain, so it's a very verdant place. That said, it's best to go when it's drier, so aim to head there between May and October. Be warned, however, that Europeans generally take their holiday in August, so the city might be very crowded at that time. San Sebastian's beautiful coasts, meanwhile, are great for a beach holiday. And it would be remiss of me not to mention Biarritz, a favorite holiday destination in the French Basque Country that is just 30 minutes away. But in spite of the proximity, you can see that there is a distinctive cultural diversity between the two.

All of these restaurants are quite expensive; the cost depends on the drinks you choose. As a rule of thumb, you're likely to pay 200 euros per person, excluding alcohol. And to ensure you get maximum enjoyment, it's best to go to these places by taxi; that way, you don't have to worry about parking or driving under the influence.

FOR STARTERS: AKELARRE

Let's get our San Sebastian tour underway at Akelarre, which is about 15 minutes out of town. Located on a hill that gives it a panoramic view of the ocean (so it's the place to be to watch the sunset and the full moon), this modern restaurant has seating for 50-55 people. Akelarre takes it first reservations for 8 p.m.

Akelarre's chef is Pedro Subijana, while his 35-year-old daughter also works as a manager at the restaurant.

Akelarre is closed in February and in the first half of October. During the week, it is also closed on Sunday evenings and Mondays. It is possible to eat à la carte, while it also has a few gastronomical menus – the latter of which might be a good idea if you want to try more than one dish. What's more, they can change some of the food in the gastronomical menu if there's anything you don't like. Akelarre serves a lot of Spanish wines, although not a lot of foreign brands. And you should especially make your way to Akelarre by taxi, as the road is windy and unlit – two things that don't mix well if you've had a drink.

SPAIN'S FIRST THREE-STAR RESTAURANT

Next on the list is Arzak. Paquita Arzak established the restaurant in the 1960s, eventually bringing her son Juan Mari Arzak on board to work in the kitchen. Now 70, Juan Mari runs the show today, along with his daughter. Arzak got its first Michelin star in 1974, its second in 1978 and its third in 1989, making it the first three-star restaurant in Spain.

When Ferran Adria became famous 10 years ago, everybody lined up to criticize him for serving 30 to 40 portions. Juan Mari, however, called up Ferran and asked to see what he was doing. After observing Ferran's work, Juan Mari said he had learned a lot from El Bulli's master and duly invited him to come to San Sebastian.

Soon, the two gastronomic titans became close friends, traveling to different places around the world together and trying different food. Their close friendship notwithstanding, they have different styles and tastes.

Juan Mari Arzak's daughter, Elena, graduated from culinary school in Sweden before becoming the restaurant's head chef. An energetic woman, Elena manages 30 people, welcomes the customers and even decides on the decoration. She is also a close friend of Mehmet Gürs of Mikla fame in Istanbul.

Scoring a reservation, however, is a tall task, so it was with Mehmet Gürs' intervention that I managed to find a table at Arzak. While enjoying my remarkable meal there, I also had the chance to see their kitchen.

Arzak is a complete Basque restaurant, although others in the area have become international. There is also one restaurant called Mugaritz that is recommended by my dear friends Vedat Milor and Mehmet Gürs, but I didn't get the chance to go. Next time I'm in San Sebastian, however, it is definitely at the top of my list.

Arzak has two gastronomical menus, both of which mainly have meat instead of fish. I managed to get half portions for each of the courses, which allowed me to try 10 portions that actually amounted to two starters, a main course and a dessert over three-and-a-half hours. Needless to say. The food and presentation were excellent.

The wine menu is also a bit more international than Akelarre's. And as for timing, I would suggest going there for dinner, since the place doesn't have an outside view.

And as a parting gift, they gave me a signed copy of a book by Juan Mari. I just need to learn Spanish first to read it…

THE THREE-STAR MARTIN BERASATEGUI

The third restaurant takes its name from its 50-year-old chef, Martin Berasategui. With its mesmerizing view of the forest, it's the perfect place to go for lunch. The restaurant is also quite modern and features a terrace during the summer.

But it was perhaps Berasategui's details that impressed me the most. For the first time ever, I saw packaged toothbrushes and toothpaste in the restroom – something that is very useful for customers. The waiters also speak English fluently, as well as many other languages.

SÃU PAULO

It's a massive city that mirrors its country's soul. The metropolis – São Paulo – might have more than its fair share of traffic mayhem and some other disagreeable characteristics, but few places are better for a holiday. When the inhabitants of the Northern Hemisphere are rubbing their hands together in a bid to stay warm during the long winter months, São Paulo offers a perfect escape for those in need of a dose of summer. There's sun, sea and sand – not to mention some great restaurants.

Here, then, are a few suggestions for your next trip to sophisticated São Paulo.

There are a number of reasons why you'd want to frequently hit the road; top of your list might be the chance to sample some great cuisine and add new discoveries to what you've tried before. Another might be the desire to head somewhere warm when the cold reigns at home. Of course, when it's winter in a northern place like Turkey, it takes a long time to reach a warm southern climate like São Paulo, Brazil's largest city. Long though the road from Turkey may be, there is one advantage: Turkish Airlines flies to the city directly every day. You board at about 10.30 in the morning, and 14 hours later, you arrive in São Paulo – with extra hours in your pocket due to the time difference.

The city has two hotels that are worth a stay. One of them is the Intercontinental, a top-quality establishment that I stayed in for a decent price. What's more, the place has a great roof lounge on the 20th floor. And if you happen to be a member of the

Intercontinental, you can enjoy breakfast, lunch and dinner at the hotel for free; if not, you'll have to shell out for the privilege. In the main, the hotel restaurants serves up a combination of Brazilian and Mediterranean fare.

Perhaps one of the best things about the Intercontinental is the fact that it's built a meter above the road. Let me explain: come the summer months of January, February and March, São Paulo gets shorts bursts of heavy rain – to the extent that the roads suddenly become rivers. If the hotel happened to be the same on the same level as the street, inundation would be inevitable. In such a situation, the hotel would lose power, the restaurant on the bottom floor would have to bail out the flood water and the elevator would be out of service; in short, the hotel would be in a lot of trouble.

Such problems are unfortunately a fact of life at the second hotel that I recommend in São Paulo, Fasano. Nevertheless, Fasano is the city's most luxurious and expensive hotel. In the past, I've happily stayed at Fasano's hotel in Rio de Janeiro; I intended to do the same in São Paulo, only to be obliged to switch to the Intercontinental after learning about the possibility of flooding at my first choice.

I did head to Fasano's restaurant for dinner one night, but lo and behold, the warnings came true: When I got there, a heavy downpour had created localized flooding that inundated the restaurant. Hotel staff brought me to another nearby restaurant owned by the chain, but I can't say that it was as exceptional as Fasano. Still, given how much I enjoyed the food at the Fasano in Rio, I was determined to dine at its São

Paulo branch as well. In the following days, I duly found a chance to grab lunch at Fasano, and it's a good thing I did; in fact, you could say the Italian hotel and its restaurant were fantastic, as the risotto and the pasta were out of this world. At both branches, they serve mozzarella di bufala – quite how they acquire the buffalo dairy product is beyond me. Now, of course, you could be right in asking why I opted for Italian cuisine in Brazil; however, if you're not going to have grilled meat, there's not much in the way of Brazilian cuisine to dig into. That's why it might just be best to go wherever your palette leads you, no matter what country you're in.

A PLACE WORTH A VISIT

But let me mention three other restaurants in São Paulo, one of which is D.O.M., a wonderful place with two Michelin stars. Until a few years ago, D.O.M. had succeeded in cracking the top 10 of the world's 50 best restaurants, but it's since lost a bit of its magic to fall into the 20s. In truth, the chef is a bit of a know-it-all. As the restaurant began to fall down the rankings, managers started to pay closer attention, but it wasn't enough to prevent the loss of a Michelin star, bringing the place down to two.

The chef only cooks on Fridays and Saturdays; on other days of the week, his assistants handle the task. D.O.M. is laid out in an open-kitchen concept, which offers diners the enjoyable prospect of surveying all the hustle and bustle that goes on in the kitchen. But regardless of who's cooking, you can't return home without trying the tasting menu. They also offer a vegetarian menu, but no matter what you're planning on having, they'll be sure to offer you some ants dried in the oven. If you ask me, though, it's a bland, tasteless and completely pointless dish! It was only out of necessity that I had this food, whose taste is similar to dried pumpkin or sunflower seeds.

Six years ago, at a time when it still had three Michelin stars, I ate a most enjoyable meal at D.O.M. And although I can't quite say I enjoy its latest incarnation, it's still a place you have to visit if you've come all the way to São Paulo. D.O.M. has three or four menus set at different prices – if you choose the smallest one, you can get a sense of what the restaurant's food is all about. There's no need, though, to try the tasting menu for wine. Instead, plump for a Chilean or Argentine wine from the wine menu.

And one final note: Because D.O.M. only seats about 40 people, it's tough to find a place to sit.

THE BEST OF THE REST: MANÍ AND JUN SAKAMATO

If you ask me, the place you really need to go to into São Paulo is Maní. They actually serve a set menu, but given that you get to select your entrée, main course and dessert, you basically get to choose your own menu. The portions are generous, so if you go as two people, I would suggest you choose different dishes – that way, you'll have a better chance to taste just some of what Maní has to offer.

Maní starts its service at the relatively late hour of 20.45 – meaning that if you're there before 20.15, you'll be confronted by a closed door. Maní also has a pleasant waiting area where you can sip a drink and place your order for your food as you wait. The fare is well worth the wait; it's only a matter of time before Maní receives a second Michelin star – or even until it enters the list of the world's 50 best restaurants. In fact, you might even say that Maní is worth a trip to São Paulo in and of itself – a mantle that it's wrested away from D.O.M.

But there's another restaurant in São Paulo that demands a visit: Jun Sakamoto, a Japanese restaurant with one Michelin star. If you go, make sure you sit at the sushi bar, lest you miss out on the show the Japanese chefs put on while preparing your meal. And just like restaurants in Japan, Jun Sakamoto doesn't use any avocado in its meals – a lesson I once learned when I was at a three-star Japanese restaurant in Japan. When I was halfway down the menu, I blurted out to the cook, "Don't you have any avocado?"

The cook seemed none too pleased at the inquiry. "Go to America," he responded in broken English. Worried about a similar chastening, I avoided even thinking about the broaching the subject in São Paulo.

Jun Sakamoto's owner must have gone to Italy at some point, as the menu even includes fresh black truffle. I really have no idea how they found the truffles, but perhaps it grows in some places in South America. Jun Sakamoto serves up some excellent grated black truffle and half-cooked sashimi. If you're in São Paulo, you just have to saddle up to the bar at Jun Sakamoto, which offers a wide sake and wine menu to boot.

If, however, you've come to São Paulo for more than four nights and have tried each of Fasano, D.O.M., Maní and Jun Sakamoto, why not try a popular place close to your hotel for your other nights in the city?

THE BEAUTIFUL ISLAND: ILHABELA

Located just over 200 kilometers from São Paulo, Ilhabela is Brazil's biggest island. Similar in size to Rhodes, Ilhabela is ringed by sandy beaches on three full sides; only the fourth side is rocky. The trip from São Paulo takes up to three hours (or two hours if your car is particularly fast – or just half an hour if you're really well-heeled and you have a helicopter). Unsurprisingly, it's a summer haunt for São Paulo's wealthy.

If you're intent on coming, here's a tip: Come on a Sunday evening and stay until Wednesday – otherwise, you'll hardly have room to move. It's impossible to find a place at a hotel or a restaurant and just as hard to find a spot to lay down your towel on the beach due to the throngs of people. From Sunday evening to Thursday morning, though, Ilhabela is far more serene, meaning there are fewer crowds to detract from your holiday.

I, indeed, did opt to come Sunday to Wednesday; while on the island, I stayed at DPNY Beach, one of the best hotels in the area. Located smack dab on the beach, DPNY also has a great Italian restaurant on site that's so good, you'd think you've gone to Italy. But if you're not in the mood for Italian, DPNY also serves up some dishes that carry a hint of French cuisine as well.

And Ilhabela isn't all just about the beach. You can take a tour around the island in a gullet or a speedboat or go on an adventure with a 4x4 jeep in the island's forested interior. If you opt for a jeep trip into the forest, make sure to lather yourself up with insect repellant, or you might not have a particularly enjoyable time.

As for me, though, I couldn't bring myself to leave that heavenly hotel to squeeze in beside dozens of others for a ride on a boat or a trip in a jeep. Even if you just stay at a hotel like DPNY, you can be sure that you'll have an extraordinarily good time simply enjoying the light waves of the sea as you survey the Brazilian mainland in front of you.

VISIT THE MUSEUM – AND FILL YOUR STOMACH

São Paulo is home to two modern art museums that deserve a visit, the Modern Art Museum of São Paulo and the Museum of Contemporary Art. What's more, both feature restaurants that offer great lunches.

SAVE YOURSELF SOME BOTHER: TAKE UBER

Traffic is a fact of life in São Paulo, as is security. That's why the best thing to do in terms of transport is to dispense with a taxi and just go for Uber – you'll be happy you did.

SYDNEY

At a time when fall is beginning to show its true colors in our – northern – part of the world, spring's just getting started in the southern hemisphere. So why not pack up and head to Australia? Who could say no to a chance to see Sydney, try some amazing food in some amazing restaurants and sip some wonderful Australian wines? And a bonus: There are all the fantastic beaches…

I had never been to the Australian continent before, but a few months ago, I made the decision to finally go for a trip. To be frank, after seeing the life there, I really regret not going before. Sydney is a terrific city whose coastal crowds and bridges carried echoes of San Francisco and Istanbul for me. When you sit on the shore, it's easy to see most of the other side. It's a city that shows two sides: There's the beauty of the view by night, and then there's the completely different beauty of the view by day. And of course, everyone already knows about the city's icon and modern architectural marvel, the Sydney Opera House. I absolutely loved Australia, and I can honestly say that, if I were to come to the world once more, I'd want to be born in Sydney.

Because modern Australia only has a history of around 200 years, there's no sign of the "historical monuments" that we are used to – what you would call a "must see" place is 160 years old at most. But set among all this newness is Sydney and its beauty. Perhaps the thing about Sydney that grabbed my attention the most was the fantastic beaches that surround the city. Wherever you are, a beach – and the accompanying chance to go for a swim – are never more than three to five minutes away by car of 15 minutes by bicycle. From October to May, when the Northern Hemisphere goes into the doldrums of fall and winter, the Australian continent enjoy spring and summer. The beaches are wonderful, while the oceans are deep-blue and clean as be; in fact, it seems that they're almost beckoning you to come. For those more used to seas as their go-to body of water, the ocean might be a bit intimidating, but don't worry, it's perfectly fine. And when you remember that it's winter or fall back home, it's eminently wonderful to jump into the water at such a time. (You certainly can't take a dip in the Atlantic in Portugal, Spain, Britain or France at the same time – you'd freeze to death.) And while Australia is known for its surfing, there are other inviting beaches where the water is almost pool-like because of breakwaters – and there's no worries about sharks to boot.

The whole place is pervaded by an atmosphere in which people constantly seem to be on holiday, only going to work when they tire of the sea and sun. It's a place where the prices are more than reasonable. Michelin doesn't publish a guide for Australia, but that doesn't mean that there aren't expensive restaurants here. Apart from these, however, you shouldn't steer clear of other excellent restaurants where you can also sample delightful food. For one, Australia is a place where you can find any type of cuisine. More than that, everything is extremely fresh and abundant; the variety of seafood is also out of this world, while agriculture is also highly developed. When you look at it, Australia is actually as big as Europe, but with just a fraction of the population, meaning there's more enough to go around for everyone. The people, too, are cheerful and social – if you happen to make eye contact with someone on the street, they'll immediately say hello. Ultimately, Australia has a profoundly easygoing nature to it that immediately seeps into your bones – especially if you're wanting to escape from the cold winter months in the Northern Hemisphere.

But of course, it would be impossible to come here and not sample some of the excellent food on offer. And in terms of choosing where to go, there could be no better advice than that of Mehmet Gürs, a chef whose Mikla in Istanbul has been named one of the world's 100 best restaurants for years (it's risen to number 44, to be exact). Like many of the chefs on the list, Gürs has been invited to showcase his skills in other countries; and because Australia has frequently come calling in his case, Gürs has cooked food at award-winning restaurants in Melbourne and Sydney (although I wonder if his interest in surfing also has something to with his selection of these restaurants). In any case, he knows every one of the Australian restaurants on the top 100 list, having cooked at them all. Furnished with his recommendations, we set off to dine, making our reservations – sometimes of our own accord and sometimes with his assistance.

So let me share a bit about these restaurants – presented, as always, in alphabetical order. And if you happen to have your own thoughts or experiences about these places, send them to me by email at metinar@metinar.com.

Without further ado, here is my list of the most

enjoyable restaurants in Sydney.

AUTOMATA

Automata is located about 15 to 20 minutes outside the city in an area that's largely home to university students. The street features about 20 or 30 restaurants in close proximity to each other in area where students meet, enjoy a drink (alcoholic or otherwise), converse, have fun or just plain hang out. Automata is a two-floor establishment that sits 50 people and serves both lunch and dinner, although the prices are the same for both. The eatery, which also has an open kitchen, boasts an easygoing atmosphere in which you eat your food at long, shared wooden tables. There are set menus for both lunch (three to five courses) and dinner (five to seven courses). There might not be any alternative to the set menu, but they do have a different set menu every day and often offer international fare and fusion dishes. The prices are also extremely reasonable. At the same time, Australian wines are quite famous – as you are no doubt aware. It's something that you really see at Automata, where you'll be spoiled for choice among the many excellent wines. The best thing at the restaurant is that they serve wine by the glass, meaning you get a chance to try many of the diverse number of wines they offer.

Because we arrived in Australia early in the morning, we elected to combine our breakfast with lunch, enjoying a three-course meal on Automata's lower floor. The fish and vegetable dishes that we had were quite light (after all, we had to think about dinner later), while we topped our meal off with a glass each of unfiltered Australian wine – white, of course. But if

I come again, my mission would be to try Automata's seven-course dinner...

BENNELONG

Bennelong is located within that most Australian of symbols, the Sydney Opera House, a masterpiece that evokes shells and includes concert, opera and theater halls. One of the shells that overlooks the city belongs to Bennelong, giving the restaurant 15-meter-high ceilings and an impressive ambiance.

The lights of Sydney, the beauty of the city's Bosphorus-style port area and the main bridge add even more to the atmosphere. Between 8 and 10 p.m., however, it's a tall order trying to find a place to sit at Bennelong. Along with some friends, I planned to have something to eat at the restaurant before heading to a concert elsewhere in the opera house – that's why we started at 6, enjoying a menu featuring a starter, main course and dessert. And in sampling what everyone else in the group had, we got a better idea about what Bennelong's kitchen is all about. If, however, you happen to come for dinner between 10 and 12, it might be better to go with the à la carte menu. In addition to Australian wines, Bennelong also serves wines from around the world – all of which are contained in a wine menu that's as thick as a telephone book. Consumed in the company of an excellent Australian wine and a breathtaking view, our meal here was easily the best I had on the continent. The ambiance was superb, as was the service. It was an evening that will live long in the memory, in part thanks to the wide menu, table layout, wine glasses, presentation, serving dishes and attentions of the three sommeliers. And even then, despite all this elegance, the price was more than reasonable. Of course, your bill might come a bit more "padded" depending on the wine you choose…

CONCRETE JUNGLE

Concrete Jungle is a very basic and plain restaurant. Set on the same street as Automata, Concrete Jungle is a breakfast place whose seating arrangement spills out onto the street somewhat. Naturally, we went for breakfast, but we also had a chance to cast an eye over its lunch and dinner menus, which are mostly vegan. It's clear to all concerned that healthy eating is at the forefront of Concrete Jungle's concept, what with its chia pudding, omelets made with egg whites, oat varieties, fruit and vegetable juices and different types of coffees. Ultimately, in the most famous of Sydney breakfast spots, we enjoyed a rather fine and healthy meal. I went for a hazelnut chia pudding decorated with banana, kiwi and papaya, as well as an omelet with egg whites, avocado, dried tomatoes and goat cheese. After that, it was time for dessert; in my case, an açai pudding with grated coconut. My daughter, on the other hand, opted for coconut juice served in a full coconut before eating the fruit itself. More than that, the bill for these mostly vegan delights wasn't even that high, totaling much the same as it would back home in Istanbul's Cihangir neighborhood.

ESTER

About 20 minutes out of town is a fantastic place for dinner, Ester, which features wooden tables and an easygoing vibe. This was abundantly clear from the fact that we had to wait for our table even though we arrived in time for our reservation. I do really wish that they had had a bar in the corner for those having to wait for their table. In the end, however, we were able to sit at a nice table, and order from the à la carte menu. And, as always, we sampled some of each other's food for a great dinner that included (for me) shellfish and Kobe steak (for my daughter). Ester only serves Australian wines. Still, they do offer a wide list with normal and organic wines and serve by the glass. In terms of price, it's a more inexpensive place that fits somewhere between Istanbul and Paris.

FISH MARKET

You can reach Sydney's fish market, which opens bright and early at 5 in the morning and closes at 5 in the evening, by either car or, on the weekends, ferry. It's a covered fish market that resembles many similar markets around the world, but that's where the similarities end. That's because there's a place to cook your fish next to every fish seller. That means you can buy your fresh fish and take it home or you can dig into a cooked version right there. Best of all, however, you can choose a combination of fish and get them to cook it right in front of you. There's no seating at the market, but you can perch at the bar – something that doesn't detract from the eating experience.

About 90 percent of the fish on sale here is local seafood, and you'll understand whether it's an import from the attached label. Ultimately, all of Sydney's fish flows through here; it's where all the hotels, restaurants and inhabitants procure their fish from. Of course, the earlier you come (it's also less crowded on a weekday), the more choice you'll have. The early bird, for instance, will have his or her choice of marinated fish, sashimi or sushi. Really, the market spoils you for choice. My favorite was the langoustine, a kind of small lobster, which was great on the grill. In the end, these kinds of places are a godsend, but more than that, the prices are good.

ORGANIC WINE THE FLAVOR OF THE DAY

Organic wines are a big thing in Australia. In organic winemaking, no sulfur – or very little of it – is added to the wine. Naturally, such wine doesn't last or age well, meaning it must be consumed in one or two years. At the same time, no sulfur means no headache! And because some wines are even made unfiltered, you can even see the particulates in the liquid. As you would expect, it's an acquired taste, but Australia provides the perfect atmosphere to try. The well-regarded Automata offers a wide selection of organic wines.

SEAFOOD OR MEAT?

The quality of the fish on offer at Australia's restaurants comes as no surprise, as the country features many delicious types of seafood that are less than common in the Northern Hemisphere. Australians make fantastic lagos and cod filets that are just right for the Turkish palette. Crayfish, shrimp and lobster are all abundant and eminently delicious. I happened to be in the country during winter, so oysters were right in season, and I certainly wasn't going to pass up the opportunity to enjoy them. At the same time, meat is not in short supply. Apart from local meat, you can sample variations on Kobe beef – an opportunity made possible by Australia's relative geographic proximity to Japan.

DON'T MISS A CONCERT IN THE OPERA HOUSE

The Sydney Opera House is truly a marvel of modern architecture. And if you take me up on my suggestion to have a meal at Bennelong, it'll be easy to head for a concert as well. The big concert hall seats about 3,000 people and has a unique design and seating arrangement. In all, about 2 million people come every year to the Opera House to view around 3,000 performances.

TAORMINA

As far as beach destinations go, Taormina is ancient. Located on the east coast of Sicily, Taormina was formed on a hill overlooking the Mediterranean 2,500 years ago, which means, of course, that is in possession of a fantastic ancient theater that sits a good 3,000. Closer to the water, however, it also has a long, beautiful beach that affords one a great chance to swim come summer.

But looming over the town is something else: Mount Etna, one of Europe's most powerful active volcanoes. On any given day, you have a good chance of seeing it puff a little bit of smoke. Heading for a visit, volcanic activity permitting, is a great way to remind yourself about just how powerful nature can be.

You need at least a week to visit Sicily; two or three days are just not enough to see Taormina and the other cities in the vicinity. The nearest airport to Taormina is in Catania, which is located to the south of Taormina, on the other side of Etna. (Catania shows many traces of the volcano's power, as it was completely destroyed by lava in 1700. In fact, there are some buildings in town in which only the roof remains visible after lava inundated the rest of the structure.)

Taormina is an exceptionally touristy place, so I suggest you not visit during the height of the season in July and August, particularly on weekends. Some say that Taormina is so crowded in these months that they hardly bother going out, preferring just to spend their time in their hotel rooms. I, for one, went in May, but even, it was still crowded.

Seeing all that Sicily has to offer is probably easiest in the company of a tour guide that can be arranged through a tourist agency. A group of eight of us went through a good agency called Legendary Sicily, which is owned by an Italian man named Eddy, a life-long tour guide who knows everything from A to Z about the area's history and geography. Packing into Eddy's jeep, we saw everything there was to see on Etna and in the 2,500-year-old town of Siracusa, which lies toward the southern tip of Sicily, from dawn till dusk.

Etna is approximately 3,500 meters high, although we climbed only about 2,000 meters of the mountain in Eddy's jeep. At one point, there is a one-kilometer-wide and 50-meter-deep channel that was formed by a past lava flow. The black volcanic rocks left behind by the flows have been a boon to the surrounding towns, particularly for the construction industry; even the shower bath of our hotel in Taormina was made from this black rock. As we clambered about on the lava flow, Eddy noted that he had seen molten lava flowing in the area 19 years ago.

The nature of the lava flows created caves that are as deep as three or four kilometers and seven or eight meters high. Walking in them with our flashlights, it was as if they had been created by humans.

All this activity, however, was more than a little tiring, so if you only have two or three days in Sicily, I suggest you first drop by Siracusa on your way from Catania's airport before heading later in the day to Taormina; though you might not get to the latter until the evening, there will be more than enough chance to see Taormina on the second day. And if you have enough time (like five hours) before any flight from Catania on the third day, you can then go and see Etna. After that, grab a late lunch in Catania and peruse the city, which is located a mere 10 minutes from the airport.

HISTORY AND NATURE ABOUND
Siracusa is home to a semi-circle Greek theater from around 500 BC, from the time when the Mediterranean basin was under Greek hegemony, as well as a full-circle Roman amphitheater from around 300 BC. Both these mesmerizing wonders of engineering and architecture are located within walking distance of Siracusa.

Another intriguing things about this ancient city is the stone quarries from 2,000 year ago. Long ago, the Roman Empire – or, more precisely, thousands of slaves – opened a hole that was 10 meters wide, 25 meters long and 100 meters deep to extract all the stones necessary for all the empire's monuments. Truly, it is amazing to imagine how they could have managed all this work. Later, Roman emperors decided to use the cave created by the quarry as a prison.

There is also another 2,500-year-old Greek monument with columns in the center of Siracusa. The structure was deformed after the emergence of Christianity in the region, and locals ultimately built walls around the columns, transforming it into a splendid church.

Siracusa is also a good place for shopping, while there are a lot of fancy restaurants near the seaside.

METROPOLE TAORMINA

For our stay in Taormina, a number of locals suggested that we stay at San Domenico, a nice place with a nice garden and view, but alas, a place that has not been renovated in years. In the end, we decided to stay at the newer Metropole Taormina – a decision we would not regret.

Located in the middle of the main street, Corso Umberto, the Metropole Taormina has 22 rooms. Though a historical building, the hotel has a modern interior design. It also boasts breathtaking views of the sea – meaning you might have some problems scoring a room in the hotel.

GRAND HOTEL TIMEO

If you can't find any room at Metropole Taormina, look no further than Timeo Hotel, a place with five stars and 70 to 80 rooms in a historical building. Even if you don't end up staying at Timeo, it's a great place to go for a drink, and perhaps even for a meal as well.

FINE DINING IN TAORMINA
TRATTORIA DA NINO

For a bite to eat, a good option is Trattoria da Nino, a simple and popular restaurant that mostly serves fish. It sits about 20 people, and has good food and wine.

RISTORANTE LA CAPINERA

Ristorante La Capinera was founded by two brothers on a location right by the water – which would especially make it the place to be on the night of a full moon. Whether for lunch or dinner, La Capinera serves up some extraordinary food. Given its excellence, it's no surprise that it requires a reservation.

The pasta in southern Italy leaves much to be desired in comparison to what's on offer in northern Italy, but the seafood is excellent in places like Taormina.

And a last word about Taormina: One simply cannot understand why there are so many churches in such a small city. So many churches, however, will afford you a chance to perhaps come across an Italian wedding.

TRATTORIA DA NINO
Address: via l. Pirandello, 37 Taormina (me)
Tel: +39 0942 21265
Website: www.trattoriadaninotaormina.com
Email: info@trattoriadaninotaormina.com

RISTORANTE LA CAPINERA
Address: via Nazionale – Spisone – Taormina Mare
Tel: 0942 626247 cell: 338 158 8013
Website: www.ristorantelacapinera.com
Email: info@ristorantelacapinera.com

METROPOLE TAORMINA MAISON D'HOTELS
Address: Corso Umberto, 154, 98039 Taormina
Tel: +39 0942 625417
Fax: +39 0942 628033
Cell: +39 329 823 6997
Website: www.hotelmetropoletaormina.it

GRAND HOTEL TIMEO
Address: via Teatro Greco 59, 98039 Taormina (me)
Tel: +39 0942 627 0200
Fax: +39 0942 627 0606
Website: www.grandhoteltimeo.com
Email: info@hoteltimeo.net

LEGENDARY SICILY TRAVEL AGENCY
Address: Salita de Luna, 10, 98039 Taormina (me)
Tel/Fax: +39 0942 620061
Website: www.legendarysicily.it
Email: legendarysicily@gmail.com

VIENNA

STEIRERECK

Located inside a city park in Vienna is Steiereck, a single-story restaurant run by a couple.

Steiereck has a tasting menu that you can order for either lunch or dinner. The restaurant can prepare the menu, one of which is fish-based and the other meat-based, depending on your preferences.

One useful thing about Steiereck is that they bring cards written in both English and German explaining the dishes – it's a great idea given that many waiters outside the United States have less than fluent English. You could even call it and ID card for the food. And if you want, you can even take the card with you when you leave the restaurant.

Steiereck offers a great view of the surrounding park thanks to its floor-to-ceiling windows, making you feel like you're eating in the center of a garden full of beautiful flowers and trees. If you're in the Austrian capital, you can do no wrong in heading to this magnificent restaurant with its remarkable dishes, presentation and design.

Note that reservations are required for Steiereck and that the place is closed on Saturdays and Sundays.

As for a place to stay, you can try Hotel Sofitel, a modern place that recently opened. It also has a nice restaurant on the top floor that you could try if you have the time.

ABOUT THE AUTHOR

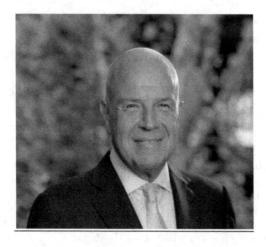

Mr. Metin Ar has been the executive chairman of the Board of Directors of Canyon Venture Partners, where he advises clients on investment banking solutions and mergers and acquisitions, since 2014. He has also been the director and chairman of the Audit Committee of Borusan Yatırım Holding, a major conglomerate with $6 billion in annual revenue, since 2014. Mr. Ar has further served as the director and chairman of the Audit Committee of the Boyner Retail Group, a non-food retail group with $1.5 billion in annual revenue, since 2015. From 2009 to 2016, he served as the chairman of Pirelli Turkey. From 2012 to 2014, he acted as the chairman of D.ream-Doğuş Restaurant Entertainment and Management. During that same period, Mr. Ar also chaired Tom's Kitchen Ltd. (UK). Earlier, he was president and CEO of Garanti Securities from 1999 to 2013. After graduating from

Bosphorus University, Mr. Ar received an M.S. in economics from the London School of Economics. The Italian government presented Mr. Ar with the Cavaliere and Grande Ufficiale medals in 2004 and 2015, respectively, for his efforts at developing Italian-Turkish bilateral commercial relations. Mr. Ar writes a restaurant blog, www.metinar.com, while he is also a discreet restaurant judge for a major culinary competition. He splits his time between Istanbul and San Francisco.